Theories, Concepts and Restructuring of Cognitive Behaviour Therapy

Theories, Concepts and Restructuring of Cognitive Behaviour Therapy

Edited by **Peter Garner**

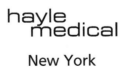

hayle
medical

New York

Published by Hayle Medical,
30 West, 37th Street, Suite 612,
New York, NY 10018, USA
www.haylemedical.com

Theories, Concepts and Restructuring of Cognitive Behaviour Therapy
Edited by Peter Garner

International Standard Book Number: 978-1-63241-366-6 (Hardback)

Contents

Preface   VII

Part 1   Theoretical and Conceptual Foundations   1

Chapter 1   Use of the Trial-Based Thought Record
to Change Negative Core Beliefs   3
Irismar Reis de Oliveira

Chapter 2   Assessing and Restructuring Dysfunctional Cognitions   29
Irismar Reis de Oliveira

Chapter 3   Modification of Core Beliefs in Cognitive Therapy   43
Amy Wenzel

Part 2   Cognitive-Behavioral Therapy   61

Chapter 4   Cognitive-Behavioral Therapy for Depression   63
Neander Abreu, Vania Bitencourt Powell and Donna Sudak

Chapter 5   Cognitive Behavioral Therapy
for Somatoform Disorders   77
Robert L. Woolfolk and Lesley A. Allen

Chapter 6   Cognitive-Behavioral Therapy
for the Bipolar Disorder Patients   105
Mario Francisco P. Juruena

Chapter 7   Cognitive-Behavioral Therapy
of Obsessive-Compulsive Disorder   127
Aristides V. Cordioli and Analise Vivan

Chapter 8   Cognitive-Behavior Therapy for Substance Abuse   145
Bernard P. Rangé and Ana Carolina Robbe Mathias

Chapter 9   **A Proposed Learning Model
of Body Dysmorphic Disorder**   159
Fugen Neziroglu and Lauren M. Mancusi

Chapter 10   **Internet Addiction and
Its Cognitive Behavioral Therapy**   171
Ömer Şenormancı, Ramazan Konkan and Mehmet Zihni Sungur

Permissions

List of Contributors

Preface

This book extensively discusses the theories, concepts and restructuring of cognitive behaviour therapy (CBT). Cognitive-behavioral therapy is the most rapidly escalating and the best factually approved psychotherapeutic approach. This book is a compilation of contributions by international veterans and aims at providing knowledge to maximum mental health professionals with updated information about CBT. It commences with an introduction of CBT and its conceptual aspects along with knowledge about the processes for assessment and restructure of cognitions. It lays stress on automatic thoughts and underlying assumptions along with the essential techniques formulated to modify core beliefs. Furthermore, the cognitive therapy of crucial psychiatric disabilities has also been discussed including reviews about the latest advances of CBT for bipolar disorder, obsessive-compulsive disability and depression. Recent developments in CBT for somatoform disabilities and latest comprehensive models for body dysmorphic disorder have also been elucidated. Towards the end, extensive details about the recent phenomenon of internet addiction and its treatment have been provided, along with CBT of the substance abuse.

All of the data presented henceforth, was collaborated in the wake of recent advancements in the field. The aim of this book is to present the diversified developments from across the globe in a comprehensible manner. The opinions expressed in each chapter belong solely to the contributing authors. Their interpretations of the topics are the integral part of this book, which I have carefully compiled for a better understanding of the readers.

At the end, I would like to thank all those who dedicated their time and efforts for the successful completion of this book. I also wish to convey my gratitude towards my friends and family who supported me at every step.

Editor

Part 1

Theoretical and Conceptual Foundations

Use of the Trial-Based Thought Record to Change Negative* Core Beliefs

Irismar Reis de Oliveira

Department of Neurosciences and Mental Health, Federal University of Bahia, Brazil

1. Introduction

The activation of certain underlying negative core beliefs (CBs) may carry out a primary role in the manifestation of cognitive, affective and behavioral symptoms. Besides aiding the patient to identify and modify dysfunctional thoughts and emotions, helping the patient to restructure dysfunctional CBs is fundamental in order for therapeutic results to be consistent and long lasting (de-Oliveira & Pereira, 2004; Wenzel, 2012). One difficulty in restructuring more superficial levels of cognition is that, frequently, the more functional alternative thoughts that are generated to challenge the dysfunctional automatic thoughts (ATs) are disqualified by thoughts (also automatic) of the type "yes, but...," derived from the activated negative CBs (de-Oliveira, 2007).

There have been several techniques developed to change dysfunctional CBs. For a review of those more commonly used, see chapter on modification of CBs in this book (Wenzel, 2012). In this chapter, I will review a novel approach to changing beliefs, namely, the Trial-Based Thought Record (TBTR; de-Oliveira, 2008; de-Oliveira, 2011d) or, in short, "The Trial."

2. Background

Although the Defense Attorney technique has been traditionally used in cognitive therapy (Freeman & DeWolf, 1992; Leahy, 2003), the Trial technique (de-Oliveira, 2008) was developed as an extension of another technique, the Sentence-Reversion-Based Thought Record (SRBTR), created to deal with "yes, but..." ATs (de Oliveira, 2007). SRBTR was mainly based on the principle that, by inverting the order of certain verbal placements containing the conjunction "but," used by the patient to disqualify his/her own accomplishments, the meaning of the sentence became more favorable and tended to change his/her mood (Freeman & DeWolf, 1992). However, some limitations, especially relative to SRBTR's implementation outside the therapist's office as homework, made its utilization difficult (de-Oliveira, 2011e).

The Trial evolved to fill in this gap, having received its name for two reasons: on the one hand it involves a simulation of a law trial, and, on the other hand, it was inspired from the work by the same name, "The Trial," by the Czech writer, Franz Kafka (1998, first published

---

*The word "negative" here does not intend to have a judgmental connotation; it means that the belief is unhelpful or dysfunctional, but in certain circumstances, "negative" CBs are helpful and functional.

in 1925). In this book, the character, Joseph K., for unrevealed reasons, is detained by law officials, and ultimately condemned and executed without ever being allowed to know for which crime he was accused (de-Oliveira, 2011e).

Starting with the idea that Kafka was perhaps proposing self-accusation as a universal principle (de-Oliveira, 2011b), which is often implicit and out of awareness, and, therefore, does not allow for an adequate defense, this technique hypothesizes that self-accusation could be understood as a manifestation of a negative CB, when activated. Therefore, the rationale for developing the Trial would be to foster awareness on the patients' part of negative CBs regarding themselves (self-accusations). In this way, unlike what happens to Joseph K. in Kafka's novel, the idea is to stimulate patients to develop more positive and helpful CBs throughout the therapy.

Also, since its original format, the Trial has evolved as a technique designed to help patients to understand and deal with the overwhelming emotional burden produced by the activation of negative CBs. As experienced clinicians know, being overwhelmed by intense emotional reactions, and not knowing how to cope to their intensity, is one of the most troubling experiences for patients (Leahy et al., 2011).

The Trial incorporates in a structured format and sequence several techniques already used in cognitive therapy and other approaches: empty-chair (Carstenson, 1955), downward arrow (Beck, 1979; Burns, 1980), examining the evidence (Greenberger & Padesky, 1995), defense attorney (Leahy, 2003; Leahy et al., 2011), thought reversal (Freeman & DeWolf, 1992), upward arrow (de-Oliveira, 2011a; Leahy, 2003), developing a more positive schema (Leahy, 2003), and positive self-statement logs (J. S. Beck, 1995).

3. Technique description

Initially, the patient is asked to present an uncomfortable situation or problem (Table 1). Normally, this corresponds to the theme chosen by the patient for the session agenda. The therapist asks what goes through the patient's mind when he/she observes a strong feeling or emotion. This phase of the technique is designed to pursue the ATs linked to the current emotional state, and is recorded in column 1. To discover which is the activated negative CB (or one to be activated), responsible for these ATs and the current emotional state, the therapist uses the downward arrow technique (Burns, 1980; de-Oliveira, 2011a). For example, the therapist asks what the ATs that were just expressed mean about the patient, assuming they are true. The answer, normally expressed as "I am..." phrases, corresponds to the activated negative CB. In the example in Table 1, the patient expressed the belief "I am weak." The therapist then explains that the procedure (Trial) begins in a similar way to an investigation or inquiry with the aim of discovering the validity of the accusation (in this case, self-accusation) that corresponds to the negative CB. The therapist then asks how much the patient finds this belief to be true and what emotions are felt. The percentages indicating the credit that the patient gives to the negative CB and the corresponding emotional response intensity are recorded in the lower part of column 1, in the space where one reads "Initial."†

---

†The space where one reads "Final" will be filled in when the session is over, after the conclusion of the task called "Preparation for the appeal." Here one assesses how much the patient believes the negative

Columns 2 and 3 of the Trial have been designed to help the patient put together information that supports (column 2) and also information that does not support (column 3) the negative CB. Column 2 corresponds to the prosecutor's performance, where the patient is stimulated to identify all the evidence that supports the negative CB, taken as self-accusation. What is normally seen is that the patient tends to produce more ATs, generally cognitive distortions, instead of evidence. I therefore suggest that the therapist not correct the patient, because later on, during the jury evaluation (column 7), the patient will be oriented to take this aspect into consideration, perceiving that the prosecutor tends to produce predominantly cognitive distortions. The information gathered and recorded in column 2 has the objective of making evident the internal arguments that the patient uses to support negative CBs.

In column 3 (defense attorney), the patient is actively stimulated to identify all the evidence that does not support the negative CB. If the therapist perceives that the patient is bringing opinions, more than evidence, he/she can subtly suggest that the patient give fact-based examples. Although patients generally improve after the conclusion of column 3 (percentage reduction corresponding to how much they deem the negative CB to be true, and the intensity of the emotional response), some do not improve or improve very little because of a lack of credibility of the alternatives brought to challenge the dysfunctional ATs. Some patients say they believe in such alternatives only intellectually.

Column 4 (prosecutor's reply to the defense attorney's allegation) is devoted to the thoughts such as "yes, but…" that the patient uses to disqualify or minimize the evidence or rational thoughts brought by the defense in column 3, causing them to have less credit. As the example in Table 1 illustrates, by using the conjunction "but," the therapist actively stimulates the expression of other dysfunctional ATs, which maintain the negative emotional reactions and dysfunctional behaviors. The mood of the patient tends to return to the level he/she presented in column 2, during the first manifestation of the prosecutor. The therapist can then use such oscillations to show the patient how his/her mood depends on how he/she perceives the situation, positively (defense attorney's perspective) or negatively (prosecutor's perspective).

Columns 5 and 6 are the central aspects of this technique. In column 5 (the defense's rejoinder in response to the prosecutor), the patient is conducted to invert the propositions of columns 3 and 4, once again connecting them with the conjunction "but." The patient copies down each phrase from column 4 and connects it to the corresponding evidence of column 3, using this conjunction. The idea is to cause the patient to reduce the force of the dysfunctional ATs. The result is the change of perspective of the situation to a more positive and realistic one. At this time, the patient is stimulated to read each one of the inverted sentences in column 5 and record in column 6 the new meaning, now positive, brought about by this strategy used by the defense attorney. The use of the upward arrow technique starts here, the therapist asking the meaning of each inverted sentence, and stimulating the patient to go further by means of the adverb "therefore". For instance, in the dialogue

---

core belief (e.g., "I'm weak"), after its deactivation and the activation of the positive core belief (e.g., "I'm strong").

between the therapist and Maria (playing the role of the defense attorney), shown in this chapter, after inverting the sentence, Maria came with "She (Maria) was away from her job for a long time, but she has 3 college degrees." Then, she added: "It seems she's not as weak as she thought. Therefore, she's not weak."

Column 7 contains the analytical part of the Trial, presented under the form of a jury deliberation. Taking the juror's perspective, the patient answers a series of questions involving the performance of the prosecutor and the defense attorney. Although many questions may be answered by the patient as a juror (e.g., Who was most consistent? Who was most convincing? Who used more fact-based information? Was there intent on the part of the accused?), the main question to be considered is: Who had the least cognitive distortions? Here, in the majority of cases, the patients acquit themselves of the accusation, represented by the negative CB, after they identify the cognitive distortions made by the prosecutor and notice that the defense attorney made no cognitive distortions.

The credit the patient attributes to the negative CB and the intensity of the corresponding emotion are evaluated at the end of each character's performance, being recorded in the lower part of all the columns (with the exception of column 5). Such percentages demonstrate the oscillation of the patient's emotions when his/her attention is focused on negative perceptions (prosecutor) or positive ones (defense attorney).

Finally, this thought record is used to activate (or even develop) new positive CBs through the above mentioned upward arrow technique (de-Oliveira, 2007; de-Oliveira, 2011a), in counterposition to the downward arrow (Burns, 1980) used in column 1. For this, the therapist asks: "Supposing the defense attorney is right, what does this say about you?" In the example of Table 1, the patient brings up the new positive CB "I am strong."

Table 2 is the homework record that the patient will be asked to fill in, being encouraged to gather on a daily basis, during the week, the elements that support the positive CB. The homework is assigned as a preparation for the appeal requested by the prosecutor when the patient acquits him/herself of the accusation, or, more rarely, requested by the defense, when the patient does not consider him/herself innocent at the end of the Trial. Also, the patient indicates daily how much he or she finds the new CB to be true.

Table 3 was adapted to fit in two or more positive CBs, when several trials and appeals have been carried out. Notice that the time taken by the patient to do the homework will be the same, regardless of how many positive CBs he/she might be nurturing in the diary. A fact, a piece of evidence or element that supports a new positive belief may support others, and in this way the patients always keep watch over the activity of the previously restructured negative CBs that, frequently, become active again if they are outside the attention span. Therefore, this form allows patients to strengthen several new positive CBs simultaneously.

The fundamental aspect at this stage is that the patient take time outside the session to pay attention to the facts and events that support the positive CBs, and this implies that the defense attorney be chosen as an ally, regardless of whether or not the patient has been absolved at the end of each Trial.

Please, briefly describe the situation: *In session, working on her difficulty to talk with her husband about her wish to quit her job.*

1. Inquiry/Establishing the accusation (core belief)	2. Prosecutor's plea	3. Defense attorney's plea	4. Prosecutor's response to the defendant's plea	5. Defense attorney's response to the prosecutor's plea	6. Meaning of the response presented by the defense attorney to the prosecutor's plea	7. Jury's verdict
What was going through your mind before you started to feel this way? Ask yourself what these thoughts meant about yourself, supposing they were true. The answer "*If these thoughts were true, it means that I am...*" is the uncovered self-accusation (core belief).	Please, state all the evidence you have that supports the accusation/core belief that you have circled in column 1.	Please, state all the evidence you have that does not support the accusation/core belief that you have circled in column 1.	Please, state the thoughts that question, discount, or disqualify each piece of positive evidence in column 3, usually expressed as "yes, but..." thoughts.	Please, copy each thought of column 4 first, and then each corresponding evidence in column 3, connecting them with the conjunction BUT.	Please, state the meaning you attach to each sentence in column 5.	Please, enumerate a list of cognitive distortions, and make a succinct report, considering who made fewer.
Downward arrow technique:	**1.** *She's spent most of her time away from her work. [A, B]*	**1.** *She has 3 college degrees.*	**1.** *...but she was away from her job for a long time. [C]*	**1.** *She was away from her job for a long time, but she has 3 college degrees.*	**It means that:**	**Prosecutor:**
I'll disappoint my husband.	**2.** *She's not able to speak with her husband about this subject. [C]*	**2.** *She's been considered the best teacher*	**2.** *...but his doesn't make a difference; for she spends much time away from work. [C]*	**1.** *She's not as weak as she thought, therefore, she's not weak.*	All-or-nothing [A], overgeneralization [B], discounting positives [C], magnifying [D],	
He's going to think that I'm not that strong woman he met years back.	**3.** *She's dissatisfied with the work she's doing. [A]*	**3.** *She has a great relationship with them.*	**3.** *...but her daughters are going to live far away. [C]*	**2.** *This doesn't make a difference; for she spends much time away from work, but she's been considered the best teacher.*	**2.** *She's not as weak as she thinks she is, therefore, she is not weak.*	**Defense attorney:**
If the thoughts above were true, what would they mean about you?	**4.** *She went almost a whole year without driving. [C]*	**4.** *Her daughters have graduated.*	**4.** *...but this is her duty. [C]*	**3.** *Her daughters are going to live far away, but she has a great relationship with them.*	**3.** *She's a good mother, therefore, she is not weak.*	No cognitive distortions
↓	**5.** *She's gaining a lot of weight. [D]*			**4.** *This is her duty, but she's a good mother, her daughters have graduated.*	**4.** *She's a good mother, therefore, she's not weak.*	**Verdict:**
I am weak						*I am innocent of the accusation.*
I feel sad						
Now, how much (%) do you believe you are *weak*? **Initial:** 95% / **Final:** 30%	Now, how much (%) do you believe you are *weak*? 100%	Now, how much (%) do you believe you are *weak*? 70%	Now, how much (%) do you believe you are *weak*? 100%	Now, how much (%) do you believe you are *weak*? 50%	Now, how much (%) do you believe you are *weak*? 30%	
What emotion does this belief make you feel? Sadness	How strong (%) is your *sadness* now? 100%	How strong (%) is your *sadness* now? 70%	How strong (%) is your *sadness* now? 100%	How strong (%) is your *sadness* now? 65%	How strong (%) is your *sadness* now? 20%	
How strong (%) is it? **Initial:** 90% / **Final:** 20%						

Homework assignment. Preparation for the appeal: Supposing that the defense attorney's pleas are true, what does it mean about you (upward arrow technique)?

Positive core belief: *I am strong* (Please, state how much you believe in this new core belief, daily, after writing down at least three pieces of evidence that support it).

Table 1. Illustration of the Trial-Based Thought Record (Copyright: Irismar Reis de Oliveira; http://trial-basedcognitivetherapy.com).

Positive core belief: *I am strong.*

Please, write down here, daily, at least one piece of evidence supporting the new core belief. Also, please, write how much (%) you believe the new core belief in the space between parentheses

Date: (50%)	Date: (%)	Date: (%)	Date: (%)
1. I got up early and went to work, despite wanting to stay in bed. 2. I came to therapy even when I didn't want to. 3.	1. 2. 3.	1. 2. 3.	1. 2. 3.
Date: (%)	Date: (%)	Date: (%)	Date: (%)
1. 2. 3.	1. 2. 3.	1. 2. 3.	1. 2. 3.
Date: (%)	Date: (%)	Date: (%)	Date: (%)
1. 2. 3.	1. 2. 3.	1. 2. 3.	1. 2. 3.
Date: (%)	Date: (%)	Date: (%)	Date: (%)
1. 2. 3.	1. 2. 3.	1. 2. 3.	1. 2. 3.

Table 2. Appeal preparation – one-belief form (Copyright: Irismar Reis de Oliveira; http://trial-basedcogitivetherapy.com).

4. Research carried out

In the first article describing the Trial (de-Oliveira, 2008), a modified version of the seven-column Dysfunctional Thought Record (Greenberger & Padesky, 1995) was proposed to change negative CBs by way of combining a strategy involving sentence reversion (Freeman & DeWolf, 1992) and the analogy to a Law trial (Leahy, 2003). The patients (n=30) took part in a jury simulation and showed changes in their attachment to negative CBs as well as in the intensity of corresponding emotions after each step during a session (investigation, prosecutor's allegation, defense attorney's allegation, prosecutor's reply, defense's rejoinder and jury's verdict). The results of this work showed significant mean reductions between the percentage figures after the investigation (taken as baseline), after the defense allegation (p< 0.001) and after the jury verdict, from the beliefs (p< 0.001) as well as from the intensity of emotions (p< 0.001). Significant differences were also observed between the first and second defense allegations (p= 0.009) and between the second defense allegation and the jury verdict with respect to the CBs (p= 0.005) and to the emotions (p = 0.02). The conclusion was that the Trial could, at least temporarily, help the patients in a constructive way to reduce the attachment to negative core beliefs and the corresponding emotions (de-Oliveira, 2008).

Please, write down here, daily, at least one piece of evidence supporting each new core belief. Also, write how much (%) you believe the new core belief in the space between parentheses.

I am strong	I am assertive	I am lovable	
Date: 8/11/11 (80%)	(50%)	(65%)	(%)
1. *I gave several classes today.*	1.	1.	1.
2.	2.	2. *My husband invited me to go out.*	2.
3. *I talked with my husband about my plan to quit my job.*	3. *I talked with my husband about my plan to quit my job.*	3.	3.
Date: (%)	(%)	(%)	(%)
1.	1.	1.	1.
2.	2.	2.	2.
3.	3.	3.	3.
Date: (%)	(%)	(%)	(%)
1.	1.	1.	1.
2.	2.	2.	2.
3.	3.	3.	3.
Date: (%)	(%)	(%)	(%)
1.	1.	1.	1.
2.	2.	2.	2.
3.	3.	3.	3.

Table 3. Appeal preparation (two or more beliefs form). (Copyright: Irismar Reis de Oliveira; http://trial-basedcognitivetherapy.com).

A clinical trial was recently completed (de-Oliveira et al., 2011) in which the Trial was studied in 36 patients with social phobia, randomly assigned to the experimental group treated with the Trial (n= 17) and to the contrast group (n= 19), this latter group treated with a conventional model of cognitive therapy that included the seven-column Dysfunctional Thought Record (DTR; Greenberger & Padesky, 1995), associated with the Positive Data Log (PDL; J.S. Beck, 1995). Both groups received psycho-education regarding the cognitive model and types of cognitive distortions, and discussed with the therapist individualized case conceptualization structured according to Judith Beck's conceptualization diagram (1995). The objective of both treatments was to restructure the CBs in order to reduce the symptoms of social phobia. Exposure was not actively stimulated in either of the groups. When a mixed ANOVA was carried out, significant reductions were observed (P< 0.001) in both approaches on scores in the Liebowitz Social Anxiety Scale (LSAS; Liebowitz, 1987), the Fear of Negative Evaluation Scale (FNE; Watson & Friend, 1969), and in the Beck Anxiety Inventory (BAI; Beck et al., 1988). Nevertheless, the one-way ANCOVA, taking the baseline data as co-variables, showed that the Trial was significantly more effective than the contrast group in reducing the FNE (P= 0.01), and social avoidance and distress (P= 0.03). The results described above justify new studies to assess the efficacy of the Trial not only in social phobia, but also in other psychiatric diagnoses.

5. Trial demonstration session[‡]

Therapist: Good morning, Maria.

Patient: Good morning, Dr. Oliveira.

T: How are you?

P: All right.

T: We have been working on an issue that has worried you a lot. So then, last week we saw this question of your decision to stop your current activity working as a teacher.

P: That's right.

T: But this is something which is giving you much doubt; during all this psychotherapeutic process that we have gone through here, this seems to have really been your great concern, and this has been a recurrent theme, hasn't it? Could you sum up our last session and what impact it had on you?

P: Yes. As during the last session we worked on the fact that I made up my mind (and this has been very difficult for me), I thought that it was important that last week we went over the advantages and the disadvantages. But this is something I had already been doing for some time.

T: We did it a little differently last time, because you had been using, for some time now, this technique of the advantages and disadvantages, but we were able to go a little further and focus on the role of reason and emotion; this internal conflict you have (one time it seems that your head tells you something, then another time it's your feelings talking). Has this changed any?

P: No, not really.

T: And you could see that actually, at that moment, the decision was not made.

P: That's right, but, although I hadn't made up my mind, I felt between then and now a little more relieved, because the impression I had before was of being paralyzed, and I wasn't doing anything to try to resolve the situation. Now, even though I haven't made a decision yet, this is the time that (as we say) I will begin to work through some situations, doing small tasks, to get better information on what is going on around me, in order to decide some time later.

T: Of course. It's important to say that the technique is called consensual role-play[§] and that it really seems to have helped you to feel more at ease, because you didn't have any obligation to make a decision, but it would be important because of what you would be learning with the situation.

P: Right.

[‡]This is a simulated session of a patient with Maria Eduarda Guedes, PsyD. The filling in of the corresponding forms, "Trial" and "Preparation for the appeal," are in Tables 1 and 2, respectively. I suggest that the reading of this demonstration be carried out at the same time as the tables.

Step 1. Inquiry

T: Tell me something, Maria: it seems to me that during this week you are still worried about this…

P: I am.

T: What has been going through your mind regarding this question of making a decision (although you told me that it is a little less difficult than before)?

P: The main issue that comes to mind is regarding my husband. I think he is the main point, because I always get the impression that I won't do what he expects me to do.

T: Exactly. And this really has been the focus of your greatest concern?

P: Yes, because this prevents me from speaking with him. A large part of my decision to not leave (of course it also has to do with the dream I've always had of being a teacher) is also because of my concern over not disappointing my husband.

T: Ok. And at these times that you are thinking of this, that is, in how to put this to your husband, in how to talk to him about this, or even the issue of maybe disappointing him, what are the thoughts and ideas that have gone through your mind?

P: First, that I will disappoint him.

T: "I'll disappoint him." Has anything else gone through your mind about this?

P: He's going to think that I'm not that strong woman he met years back.

T: So he'll think that you aren't that strong woman he once knew.

P: Right.

T: And, if it's true (only when we start from the principle that this thought may be true), what does this mean to you?

P: That in fact I am not strong anymore… so, that I am weak.

T: Ok. Is this an idea that goes through your mind once in a while?

P: Yes! Every time I think about the idea of leaving my position as a teacher, I get this idea that I'm being weak, that I could keep on trying…

T: That's interesting, Maria, because we have talked a lot during therapy, and since the beginning (when I showed you this psychotherapy model), you could see this conceptualization diagram that seems to have helped. And what is interesting is that many of these ATs that I explained to you and that are at the first level, are often the result of the idea you have of yourself, of how you see yourself as a person, which we call…

P: Core belief.

T: Core belief, you remember very well. If we were to put this down as an activated core belief, and wrote down here "I'm weak," would this make sense to you? Can you see this as this arrow going up here, nurturing these thoughts? [Therapist points to the arrow going from the core belief box to the ATs box (Fig. 1.)]

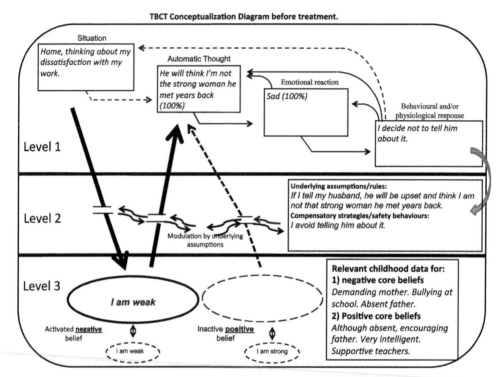

Fig. 1. Maria TBCT conceptualization diagram (Phase 1), showing the negative core belief activated more frequently before treatment.

P: That makes sense.

T: Would it be worthwhile for us to work on this idea a bit, this concept that you are presenting here, which seems to return every now and then?

P: Yes.

T: What I want to propose to you today is that we work with this by using something that hasn't been done yet in our sessions; it's a technique called "The Trial." In this technique, the central idea that people are burdened about themselves (in your case, "I'm weak") is like a type of self-accusation, it's how you see yourself, isn't that right? I'm going to write down on this form exactly this: "I'm weak;" and you saw that we had several thoughts that were written here, related, even, to the question of your husband, and the phase of this technique corresponds to what we call the investigation; and in the investigation (assuming these thoughts are true) you yourself came to this conclusion: "I'm weak." How much do you believe this, Maria ("I'm weak"), now?

P: Today, now, 100%.

T: 100%. By believing this 100% ("I'm weak"), what do you feel? What is the emotion that corresponds to this?

P: I feel sad. I've felt like this for some months…

T: "Sadness." Ok. If you had to evaluate the amount of this sadness, what would it be now (from 0 to 100)?

P: When I think that I am weak, it is 100%.

Step 2. Prosecutor's plea

T: 100% also, right? Now I would like us to follow this same line of thought (as if you were in a tribunal, a courthouse) and that, taking this as a self-accusation, I want you to prove to me that this is true, that you are weak, all right? One thing I want to ask you to do (and it's something you've already started doing in the consensual role-play technique we used last session) is to live out these internal characters. So, for example: we have several empty chairs here and in that chair over there in front (where I'd like you to sit now), you will be yourself, Maria. Can you do this? You are being placed as a defendant, and the charge is "I'm weak." When we did the investigation just a while ago, you said that you believe this very much. Do you, Maria, seated there, maintain this belief at 100% (how much do you believe it)?

P: Yes.

T: Ok. And is the sadness still high?

P: It's still at 100%.

T: Why don't you sit down in this chair? And now you will represent one of your internal characters, the one that accuses you of being weak. Can you sit down over here?

P: I think I'm good at this!

T: You're good at this, great! Ok then, you will make the charge against Maria, who is seated in that chair, and you will prove, bring the arguments that you have as a prosecutor to accuse her of being weak.

P: She's spent most of her time on leave of absence or away from her work.

T: Ok. "She's spent most of her time away from her work."

P: Right. She's not able to speak with her husband about this subject.

T: "She's not able to speak with her husband about this subject."

P: She's dissatisfied with the work she's doing.

T: Ok. So "she's dissatisfied with the work she's doing."

P: She has had more than one crisis during some classes. She went almost a whole year without driving.

T: Ok. "She went almost a whole year without driving."

P: And now, Dr. Oliveira, she's gaining a lot of weight and she can't lose it.

T: Ok. "She's gaining a lot of weight." I'd like you to go back to that chair. See what you've just heard from this character, the prosecutor, really trying to prove that you are weak, with the following arguments: You've spent most of your time away from your work; you can't speak with your husband about this subject; you are not satisfied with the work you are doing; you've already had more than one crisis during classes; and you went almost a year without driving, besides gaining a lot of weight. When you hear these arguments voiced by this character that just expressed herself, how much do you believe this ("I'm weak")?

P: 100%

T: 100%. And the sadness?

P: 100%. Can I make it 110%?

T: Ok. Actually, we can have an idea that, if it is at 100% now (and it was weaker before), maybe it wasn't at 100% before. Would you like to re-evaluate...?

P: I don't know, 95% before.

T: 95% before, and the sadness was as high as it is now?

P: It's higher now.

T: So, how much was it before, if now you consider it as being 100%?

P: 90% before.

Step 3. Defense attorney's plea

T: Ok, 90% before. Maria, once in a while, don't you give a chance to the other side (to the character that is the defense attorney) to express itself, to be manifested? I'd like you to do that now. We are in a tribunal, why don't you sit in this chair now, and answer the accusations made by the prosecutor? That is, Maria is in that chair, you have put yourself here as her defense...

P: I'm supposed to defend, right? I'm not very good at this.

T: What is interesting is that maybe your character that would be from the defense has not had much chance to express itself, and to begin with, maybe one of the great difficulties is the concept of a defense attorney. Is the defense attorney obliged to believe in the innocence of the accused?

P: No.

T: That is, everyone deserves a defense. If you had to speak about her, Maria, and defend her as your client, what arguments would you bring forth? All a defense attorney has to do is do a good job, right?

P: I'm not sure, Dr. Oliveira, if the fact that I've gotten 3 university degrees counts....

T: Ok. Is it a fact? Is it something that really speaks in favor of Maria?

P: Yes, it does.

T: That is, "she's gotten 3 degrees."

P: On the other hand, this could be considered a failure.

T: The interesting this is: who is talking now?

P: The prosecutor.

T: Is this the time for the prosecutor to speak?

P: No.

T: What is your role in this case, seated in that chair?

P: The defense.

T: Exactly, and from the defense's point of view, what will you say regarding your client? You consider this as what?

P: A fact.

T: A fact that really defends her.

P: Besides the 3 degrees, she's been considered a good teacher.

T: So, "she's been considered a good teacher..."

P: ...one of the best. Last month, we had a 'teacher week' in her city, and normally the teacher with the best performance is chosen. She was the chosen one.

T: OK. Can you bring more elements in defense of Maria?

P: She has a great relationship with her daughters, but...

T: "But..."

P: The prosecutor is speaking, and it's not her turn.

T: So, let's call attention to the prosecutor so that she will really be silent at this time, because her place is here [the therapist points to the other chair] and, when the time comes for her to speak, she will have all the freedom to do so, but, right now, she remains silent, right? So, you, as the defense attorney, would say what?

P: She has a great relationship with her daughters.

T: Any other element?

P: I think that the fact that her daughters, today, have both graduated (one is a lawyer and the other an architect) indicates that she's a good mother.

T: "She's a good mother." So, while writing this, it would be interesting to put down exactly what shows that she is a good mother, so we can put it in parentheses as a reminder.

P: The fact, right, doctor?

T: The more facts, the better.

P: Her daughters have graduated from college.

T: "Her daughters have graduated." Maria, now, I'd like you to return to that chair again, and listen to what your defense attorney has just stated. You have 3 different college degrees; You've been considered the best teacher; You have a great relationship with your daughters; You're a good mother (what proves this is that your daughters have even graduated). While listening to your defense attorney, how much do you believe this ("I'm weak")?

P: I believe it a little less... around 70%.

T: What happens to the sadness, Maria?

P: It also goes down... to 70%.

Step 4. Prosecutor's second plea

T: 70%. Now, I'd like you to return to this chair over here. This is the time the prosecutor can speak again. Would you come over here? Normally, at this time in this type of activity, the prosecutor has already used the arguments she had, and, generally speaking, what she will do is to "undo" what was said by the defense. Usually the prosecutor uses the conjunction "but," and this is what I'm going to give you the chance to do. That is, the defense attorney said: "She has 3 different degrees," but...(what does the prosecutor say?).

P: ...but she was away from work for a long time.

T: Ok. "She was away from work for a long time."

P: ...which makes her feel dissatisfied.

T: "She's been considered the best teacher," but...

P: But this doesn't make any difference, since she's away from her job so much!

T: "This doesn't make any difference, since she's away from her job so much." Ok. "She has a great relationship with her daughters," but...

P: The one she's closest to got married and lives in São Paulo.

T: And how would you sum that up?

P: They are becoming more distant.

T: "They are becoming more distant." Distant in the sense of living farther away, isn't that right?

P: Yes.

T: This is for us to have an idea of what "more distant" means...

P: ...and the other one is also getting married.

T: "They're going to live far away." "She's a good mother, her daughters have graduated," but...

P: This is her duty; make sure her kids get a college education.

T: "This is her duty; making sure her kids get a college education." Ok? Why don't you return to that chair, as Maria? And what you've just heard from the prosecutor, who was seated here, was: You were away for a long time (regarding the question of the college courses you were taking); This doesn't make any difference, since you're on leave a lot and don't work as a teacher; They are living far away (here, you are referring to your daughters); This is your duty, making sure they get a college education. While listening to your prosecutor, how much do you believe this ("I'm weak")?

P: This technique isn't helping me, because I've gone back to believing 100%: I'm a failure.

T: 100%, "I'm a failure." So it goes up. And what about the sadness, what happens?

P: It goes up as well.

T: As well, 100%. This is very important, what you've just said... – and I apologize for perhaps making you feel uncomfortable. Might this be what happens outside this office? Which voice do you listen to more outside, the prosecutor's or the defense attorney's?

P: I almost don't hear the voice of the defense attorney.

T: And the prosecutor is always speaking?

P: Yes.

T: Wasn't this what she just did? She just spoke. And what can you learn right after hearing what was said by the prosecutor (something that appears to be very frequent in your life)?

P: That I'm always blaming myself...I'm always bringing accusations against myself.

T: Doesn't it seem that way?

P: Yes.

Step 5. Defense attorney's second plea

T: Ok. So what if you did the same thing now, here in this chair (where you'll be seated as your defense attorney)... Can you do this now?

P: Yes, I can.

T: What is interesting is that you can use the same strategy used by the prosecutor; in this case you'll also use the conjunction "but." In the same way that the prosecutor didn't seem to have many more arguments than those already used, nor does the defense attorney, but the good news is that it isn't necessary. What I'd like to ask you to do now, Maria, is the following: why don't you copy down exactly what was said by the prosecutor?

P: "She was away from her job for a long time."

T: And I'd like you to add the conjunction "but" right after that.

P: "But..."

T: I'd like you to copy down exactly what was said by the defense.

P: "...but she has 3 different college degrees."

T: Can you read this sentence to me again?

P: "She was away from her job for a long time, but she has 3 college degrees."

T: What does this mean to you, as Maria's defense attorney?

P: This means that it seems she's not as weak as she thinks she is.

T: Why don't you also place a number to correspond exactly to what you just told me?

P: "This means that..."

T: "...it seems that she's not as weak..."

P: "It seems she's not as weak as she thought."

T: I'd like you to add the word "therefore" here. I'd like you to finish the sentence.

P: Therefore, she's not weak.

T: Why don't you write exactly this? It would be enough for you to just repeat this same strategy.

P: "This doesn't make a difference; for she spends much time away from work, but she's been considered the best teacher."

T: What does this mean about Maria?

P: Again, this means that she's not as weak as she thinks she is.

T: Why don't you write down exactly this?

P: "She's not as weak as she thinks she is."

T: Therefore…?

P: Therefore... she is not weak.

T: Can you do the same thing with the other one?

P: "Her daughters are going to live far away, but she has a great relationship with them."

T: What does this mean to you?

P: It means that she's a good mother.

T: Why don't you write down there exactly this?

P: Therefore… she is not weak.

T: Can you do that with the last one?

P: This is her duty; making sure that her kids get a college education, but she's a good mother, her daughters have graduated.

T: What does this mean to you?

P: It means, again, that she's a good mother.

T: Why don't you write that down there?

P: Therefore… she's not weak.

T: Maria, I'd like you to once more take your seat and say, with these facts before you or from what was just said by your defense attorney (It seems that you are not as weak as you thought, therefore you're not weak; This means that you're not as weak as you thought, therefore – once again – you're not weak; You're a good mother, therefore you're not weak; You're a good mother – again – therefore, you're not weak), facing all this, how much do you believe ("I'm weak")?

P: 50%.

T: 50%. What happens to the sadness?

P: I'm a little more relieved... 65%.

Step 6. Jury's verdict

T: 65%. Maria, here's the thing: in this phase of a tribunal, the prosecutor had a chance to speak, so did the defense; there was the rebuttal of the prosecutor; there was the rejoinder from the defense; what is the next step in a judicial process such as this one?

P: The jury's decision?

T: Exactly, the jury meets alone. What I'd like you to do now, Maria, is exactly that: could you sit in that chair and take the place of juror number 1? So, imagine yourself now gathered in a room with several people; you have all the time in the world, although here, actually, we only have a few minutes left for this. But I'd like you to picture yourself gathered with this body of jurors and that you'd leave here with a unanimous result. And I'd like to ask you as a juror, what is the role of a jury member?

P: Evaluate what was said by the prosecutor as well as by the defense attorney; weigh the facts and reach a verdict.

T: Ok. And normally these jurors would answer some questions such as: which of the two was more consistent, more convincing, was based more on facts and distorted the facts the least? And here we are speaking of cognitive therapy, so, of the cognitive distortions. Who was more concerned with the dignity of the accused? Were there any mitigating circumstances? Was there any intent? So, these are the questions that are asked when the jurors meet. I'd like you to see, in this case, how a juror really should act, therefore, with objectivity and ethics. And it would be very interesting (if you've already seen the movie "12 Angry Men") for you to picture yourself in the room with the jurors.

P: So I have to...

T: ...observe what was said by the prosecutor and the defense attorney, and the prosecutor's rebuttal, then the defense attorney again, and try to answer these questions.

P: So here the prosecutor said that she's spent most of her time away from work... I think that here - although it is true -, in the last year she returned to her job and has worked more than she's gone on leave.

T: Therefore, is there some level of cognitive distortion in that?

P: Yes.

T: From what you've already learned through our work, could you name these distortions?

P: I think overgeneralization, she's overgeneralizing here... But I can see that, besides this one, the prosecutor used very concrete facts. "She can't speak with her husband." This is a fact... about this subject.

T: Even if it's a fact, would you consider that, as a juror, there is some cognitive distortion?

P: It's not all the time that she can't talk with him; she really does talk with him about many things, but regarding this subject she hasn't been able to.

T: So you could see that, according to the prosecutor, the fact of not being able to speak with him indicates that she is weak. What conclusion do you reach from this?

P: That the prosecutor was heavy handed.

T: Ok.

P: "She's not satisfied with the work she does." This is a fact. People can say this or that regarding her classes, but long ago she got pleasure from what she did; today she doesn't, so this is a fact.

T: Ok. If you take into consideration that all those questions (mitigating circumstances, intent, a series of other things on which a juror really bases himself on), is this enough to accuse her of being weak or would you say that there is a problem with that?

P: No, it isn't enough. It's a fact, it's true, but in and of itself it doesn't make her a weak person. "She's had several crises in classes." This is real and it makes her a weak person. But, with regard to the defense attorney, the elements stated were really very damaging, even convincing. So, "she has 3 degrees"... Although, Dr. Oliveira, every time I think of this I get the impression that I was never able to stick with any of the courses...

T: Ok. Which character are you incorporating right now?

P: The prosecutor.

T: But you are there as a juror, even to hear the prosecutor, right?

P: So I guess the defense attorney did a good job here.

T: Is there any distortion, something not based on facts?

P: No, it's true. "She's been considered a good teacher," that is real. "She has a great relationship with her daughters," this is very true. "She's a good mother"... I don't think that the fact that her two daughters graduated from college is an indication of her being a good mother.

T: And are you speaking now as the prosecutor, the defense or the juror?

P: I think as the juror; I'm denying what the defense said.

T: Ok. The interesting thing is that, strictly speaking, you are taking only one aspect into account, right? And a juror will analyze many aspects. And when you analyze all this as a juror, even upon seeing the other points stated by the prosecutor and the defense attorney...?

P: The elements the defense attorney brings me have more weight.

T: OK. Would you say that you are close to reaching a position of unanimity, considering that context we cited, to give the verdict?

P: Yes... the verdict is that she's innocent.

T: Why don't you write that down exactly?

P: ...since the proof the defense attorney brings is more convincing. I think that's it.

T: So why don't you return to that chair, Maria? You heard the juror that brought this result, this verdict that considers you innocent of this accusation brought by the prosecutor. At this time, how much do you believe this ("I'm weak")?

P: It's still there, but the way I believe it is weaker... so I guess it's around 30%.

T: 30%. What is happening to the sadness now, how big is it?

P: It's a lot more reduced, at 20%.

Step 7. Preparation for the appeal

T: 20%. What we could do now, Maria, is precisely a question that is extremely important. You've just heard all these internal characters; would you say that the prosecutor, upon receiving the result that she lost at this time, is going to be satisfied, or will something make her speak out?

P: Always, she'll always want to speak out.

T: What way will she speak out?

P: Raising more issues.

T: So, it seems to me that she is asking for an appeal... and we will give her this appeal. That is, as many times as it is necessary, we'll return to this tribunal. If the defense had lost, we'd also give it the possibility of an appeal. Ok, but there is a very important choice for you to make now: who do you choose as your ally? The prosecutor who was seated in that chair, or the defense attorney?

P: The defense attorney.

T: If the defense attorney is right in having you acquitted now, if the juror is right in giving you this verdict, what does this mean about you, Maria?

P: If the defense attorney is really right? This proves that I'm not weak.

T: Therefore you are...

P: I still wouldn't say that I am strong...

T: Ok. Whose voice would you say – even if you don't yet affirm it – that you are trying to listen to?

P: The defense attorney's.

T: The defense? Saying that you are still not that strong?

P: No, no, the prosecutor's!

T: The prosecutor's. And who are you choosing as your ally?

P: The defense attorney.

T: This attorney who was seated here, with all those arguments, did she at any time doubt that you were innocent? No. Therefore, what would the defense attorney say, if she were in your place?

P: She'd say "I am strong."

T: Why don't we give credit to the defense attorney, who was so absent and had so little opportunity to speak? And if we wrote down on this other document... and from now on, I'd like us to sit over here at this table... here's the thing: I'd like you to prepare yourself for the appeal requested by the prosecutor. And you are placing here the very document of the defense, which I'd like to present to you. What does a good defense attorney do between hearings, when he is working on a case?

P: He continues looking for evidence and elements in favor of his client.

T: And when he doesn't find any, what does he do?

P: He continues searching.

T: He continues searching, therefore, he doesn't stay still. This means we are talking about an ethical attorney; seek does not mean forge, it means going after facts. And I have something in mind on speaking of this: what are the facts that represent who we are? Are they the heroic ones, or the small facts of our routine?

P: Although I think it's the heroic facts, rationally speaking, it's the day-to-day facts.

T: It's these facts that say who we are.

P: Yes.

T: These facts will say whether we are weak or strong. And what conclusion did your defense attorney reach?

P: That I am strong.

T: So, would you have any objection if we placed here, at least temporarily, "I am strong"?

P: Temporarily, no.

T: Even if it is temporary, would there be any possibility of you, on a daily basis and along with your defense attorney, looking for up to 3 facts that would indicate that you are strong, to help your defense attorney's performance?

P: It does take some time to do this...

T: What if we tested out this idea now? For example, if you had to think about today, would you be able to (from the time you got up) bring some elements that demonstrate this, since you came to the conclusion that we don't really need a heroic fact for such?

P: So little has happened today that I can't take anything into consideration...

T: Ok, so describe to me a little of your day so far.

P: My alarm clock went off at 7 this morning and I was still very sleepy.

T: Ok, what happened following that?

P: I got up.

T: What did you feel like doing right then?

P: Staying in bed.

T: And when you got up despite wanting to stay in bed, what did this mean?

P: That I got up… that I wasn't weak at this time.

T: Ok. So, even with this small doubt, could you write it here as an item that describes this?

P: Oh, Dr. Oliveira, it's my obligation, I have to get up and go to work!

T: Ok. And what character is speaking right now?

P: The prosecutor.

T: And the question I ask you is this: whose is this document?

P: The defense attorney's.

T: And therefore, you are allowing the prosecutor to use a document that isn't hers? Ok, it doesn't matter that the prosecutor says this. This document belongs to the defense attorney and it appears as though you decided to work with her. So, if you are working with the defense – even if you, Maria, have doubts, or don't have much desire to do so because you still don't trust your defense attorney very much – would it be possible to give her a vote of confidence by writing this down?

P: "I got up early and went to work."

T: It seems that you stated this another way, "despite…"

P: "…despite wanting to stay in bed."

T: Ok. Does this give it a somewhat different connotation? Could you state another fact? If you find it difficult, continue talking about your morning… what happened next?

P: I didn't want to come here today.

T: Ok. Was it difficult to come here today?

P: Yes, because I was already late leaving a class, I arrived here late, I thought there wouldn't be enough time, and I didn't feel like coming anyway…

T: And what did you do?

P: I came.

T: And what does this mean?

P: That… I was strong…?

T: Isn't this a small element nurturing this here ("I am strong")? And in fact, you don't need any heroic fact; you just need small elements like this one.

P: "I came to therapy even when I didn't want to"?

T: Exactly. This means that you really had to mobilize enough decision, energy and willpower, isn't that right? I'm going to leave this third item for you to do as the day goes on. Now, tell me something: seeing these two elements here and remembering the viewpoint of the defense attorney (because this is a document of the defense, and, at this time, you are representing the defense, or allying yourself to her), how much do you believe this ("I am strong")?

P: I believe it 50%.

T: Why don't you write here "50%"? You can even modify this today, if you find another element. I'd like to ask you to, each day, put the date here in this space, seek out 3 elements, and daily, evaluate how much you believe this ("I am strong").

P: All right.

T: Maria, how much do you believe the negative core belief "I'm weak" now?

P: The same: 30%.

T: And how strong is your sadness now?

P: Also the same: 20%.

T: Ok? So, what will happen, or what do you hope will happen when you arrive with this information (that you gathered to work with your defense attorney) to answer the prosecutor's request for an appeal?

P: I'll be prepared for whatever comes from the prosecutor...

T: Exactly, that is the our goal, isn't it? And maybe another goal is to work in order for your defense attorney to gain more practice.

P: That as well.

T: She has been very silent or even absent for all these months, or years... Maria, if we could go back there... and if you could now tell me what the work we did here today meant to you, what would you tell me?

P: First of all, Dr. Oliveira, I'm going to leave here today feeling a bit stronger. Not as a strong person, but a little stronger than when I arrived here. I can see now the way my defense attorney was lying dormant all this time and I think that today I began to wake her up. Maybe, starting today, and especially with practice...

T: Ok. I only want to show you this diagram again [Therapist shows phase 1 of the TBCT conceptualization diagram to the patient in Fig. 1]; what do you see happened here (now, with this work we did)?

P: That I began to activate a little more this belief that was very weak or even inactive.

T: Exactly, it's as if it were here in this space, while the other belief was quite strong (you see this arrow going up and demonstrating that, since you are weak, normally the thoughts correspond to this). What if we looked at this other diagram, would you say that what happened here was exactly that? That is, what happened to this arrow? [Therapist shows phase 2 of the TBCT conceptualization diagram to the patient in Fig. 2]

P: It doesn't activate my negative core belief (that I am weak), it directly activates the belief that I am strong...

T: Do you think it would be acceptable for us to write exactly this here: "I am strong"?

P: Yes, it would.

T: What do you imagine will happen now, while you have this positive belief "I am strong," in relation to this level that I explained to you in the beginning?

P: It is still a belief that doesn't stay activated the whole time, isn't it?

T: Ok, and would you say that it is activated now?

P: It *is* activated now.

T: And, being activated right now, what thoughts would you say are going on, in this space of ATs? [Therapist points to ATs box in the TBCT conceptualization diagram in Fig. 2]

P: ...that maybe I'll be able to deal with conversing with my husband.

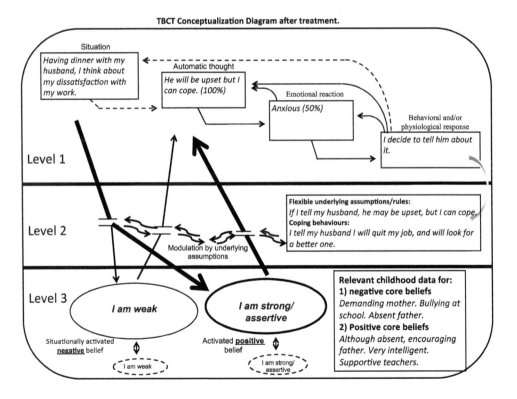

Fig. 2. Maria TBCT conceptualization diagram (Phase 2), showing the positive core belief activated more frequently after restructuring of cognitions with TBCT.

5.1 Obstacles to be avoided by the therapist when conducting a trial session

Here are some of the obstacles therapists should avoid in order to make the TBTR work optimally:

1. Make sure that sentences are relatively short so that the patient has no problem when reversing them (long sentences are difficult to understand by the patient after sentence reversal);
2. Make sure that the defense attorney's arguments are not exclusively limited to responding to the prosecutor's plea; stimulate the patient to explore different aspects and areas of his/her life (other than the accusation);
3. If you do not succeed in finishing the Trial during one session, do not stop the Trial just after the prosecutor's plea; try always to stop it after the defense attorney's plea;
4. If the patient considers him/herself guilty, this is not a problem; the defense attorney should ask for an appeal so that the Trial can be repeated in the following session as an appeal; in this case, it is essential that homework be that the patient gather evidence that confirms the positive core belief (choosing the defense attorney as an ally);
5. If the patient decides (and this is rare) that s/he will continue working with the prosecutor instead of the defense attorney for homework assignment, interrupt the Trial and ask him/her for advantages and disadvantages of such a decision;
6. When the prosecutor interrupts the defense attorney's plea with "yes, but..." thoughts, gently tell the patient that the prosecutor should wait for his/her turn; on the other hand, if the patient tends to use the defense arguments when playing the role of the prosecutor, tell him that the defense attorney should wait for his/her turn (in this case, the patient should be praised for thinking positively, but, in any case, the patient should return to the prosecutor's plea);
7. Sometimes the negative core belief is so activated that, after reversion of the sentences, the patient does not succeed in seeing or admitting the positive side shown during the second defense attorney's performance (when searching for the meaning in the reversed sentence). In this case, ask him/her: Who is speaking now? If the patient recognizes the prosecutor acting, gently ask him/her the meaning of the sentence in the defense attorney's perspective, reminding him/her that this is the defense attorney's turn;
8. Sometimes, the patient has no evidence or argument as a prosecutor against the defense attorney's plea after the therapist reads the sentence and says "but..." In this case, draw a line and, when inverting the sentences, just copy the sentence and ask the patient what it means...;
9. The meaning of the reversed sentence should never be a broad interpretation; please, encourage the patient just to say what the sentence means by itself; that is fine when the patient brings meanings like: "I am intelligent," "I am normal," "I am a good father," etc.;
10. Finally, in some severe axis I disorders and in some personality disorder patients, even when the defense attorney is repeatedly successful in acquitting the patient, self-accusation returns (negative core belief easily activated); in this case, use the Trial II (where the patient sues the prosecutor, accusing him/her of incompetence (never won a lawsuit), abuse (pursues the patient everywhere) and moral harassment

(humiliates the patient). Results are amazing and durable. This is a step when the patient is informed and trained in taking some perspective (metacognition). The prosecutor has much less or no more credibility for him/her at this stage. It is advisable that the therapist be duly trained and supervised to engage in this step (de-Oliveira, 2011c).

6. Conclusion

Dealing with negative CBs will mobilize what is most significant for the patient, and consequently carry a strong emotional charge. This procedure should be carried out with extreme care and respect. It is suggested to non-experienced therapists that they utilize the Trial, if possible, at least initially, after training and supervision.**

7. Acknowledgements

I am deeply indebted to Alessandra Mendonça Gomes and Tiana Coêlho da Gama Santos for important suggestions during the development of Trial-Based Cognitive Therapy. Their insights and comments made this approach much better than would have been possible without their help. Thanks are also due to Vania Powell – who helped me implement the studies – and to Donna Sudak and Amy Wenzel for intellectual assistance and guidance in the development of my work as a cognitive therapist.

8. References

Beck AT (1979) Cognitive therapy and the emotional disorders. New York: Meridian.

Beck AT, Epstein N, Brown G, Steer RA (1988) An inventory for measuring clinical anxiety: psychometric properties. Journal of Consulting and Clinical Psychology, 56:893-897.

Beck JS (1995) Cognitive therapy: basics and beyond. New York: Guilford Press.

Burns DD (1980) Feeling Good: The New Mood Therapy. New York: Signet.

Carstenson B (1955) The auxiliary chair technique – a case study. Group Psychotherapy, 8:50-56.

De-Oliveira IR (2007) Sentence-reversion-based thought record (SRBTR): a new strategy to deal with "yes, but..." dysfunctional thoughts in cognitive therapy. European Review of Applied Psychology, 57:17-22.

De-Oliveira IR (2008) Trial-Based Thought Record (TBTR): Preliminary data on a strategy to deal with core beliefs by combining sentence reversion and the use of an analogy to a trial. Revista Brasileira de Psiquiatria, 30:12-18. (free pdf version available at http://www.scielo.br/pdf/rbp/v30n1/a03v30n1.pdf).

De-Oliveira IR (2011a) Downward/upward arrow: Accepted entry in Common Language for Psychotherapy Procedures (www.commonlanguagepsychotherapy.org, retrieved in August 7, 2011).

De-Oliveira IR (2011b) Kafka's trial dilemma: Proposal of a practical solution to Joseph K.'s unknown accusation. Medical Hypotheses, 77:5-6.

**Information on training and supervision may be found in http://trial-basedcognitivetherapy.com/.

De-Oliveira IR (2011c) Trial-based cognitive therapy: Accepted entry in Common Language for Psychotherapy Procedures (www.commonlanguagepsychotherapy.org, retrieved in August 7, 2011).

De-Oliveira IR (2011d) Trial-based thought record: Accepted entry in Common Language for Psychotherapy Procedures (www.commonlanguagepsychotherapy.org, retrieved in August 7, 2011).

De-Oliveira (2011e) Uso do "Processo" para modificar crenças nucleares disfuncionais. In: Rangé B, Diálogo com a Psiquiatria. Artmed, Porto Alegre.

De-Oliveira IR, Pereira MO (2004) Questionando crenças irracionais. In: Abreu CN & Guilhardi HJ. Terapia comportamental e cognitivo-comportamental: práticas clínicas. São Paulo, Roca. 482 p.

De-Oliveira IR, Powell VB, Wenzel A, Seixas C, de-Almeida C, Grangeon MC, Caldas M, Bonfim T, Castro MM, de-Almeida AG, Moraes RO, Sudak D (2011) Controlled study of the efficacy of the Trial-Based Thought Record (TBTR), a new cognitive therapy strategy to change core beliefs, in social phobia. Journal of Clinical Pharmacy and Therapeutics, in press (doi:10.1111/j.1365-2710.2011.01299.x).

Freeman A, DeWolf R (1992) The 10 dumbest mistakes smart people make and how to avoid them. New York: HarperPerennial.

Greenberger D, Padesky CA (1995) Mind over mood. New York: Guilford Press.

Kafka F (1998) The trial. New York: Schocken (first published in 1925).

Leahy RL (2003) Cognitive therapy techniques. A practitioner's guide. New York: Guilford Press.

Leahy RL, Tirch D, Napolitano LA (2011) Emotion regulation in psychotherapy. New York: Guilford Press.

Liebowitz MR (1987) Social phobia. Modern problems in pharmacopsychiatry, 22:141-173.

Watson D, Friend R (1969) Measurement of social-evaluative anxiety. Journal of Consulting and Clinical Psychology, 33:448-457.

Wenzel A (2012) Modification of core beliefs in cognitive therapy. In: De-Oliveira (ed.) Cognitive-behavioral therapy. InTech, Rijeka, Croatia.

2

Assessing and Restructuring Dysfunctional Cognitions

Irismar Reis de Oliveira
Department of Neurosciences and Mental Health,
Federal University of Bahia,
Brazil

1. Introduction

Cognition impacts clinically relevant aspects of day-to-day function, such as emotion, behavior, and interpersonal relationships, and involves structures necessary to support information processing. The exchange of interpersonal information in therapy typically comprises emotional states, behavioral symptoms, expectations for improvement, and experiences and meanings attached to experiences, that may occur according to implicit (non-conscious) and explicit (conscious) levels of awareness on the part of both the client and the therapist (Alford & Beck, 1997).

This chapter has two learning objectives: 1) help the patient to identify and change cognitions in the first and most superficial level of information processing – comprising negative automatic thoughts (ATs), and expressed as consistent errors in patients' thinking; 2) help the patient to identify and change cognitions in the second and intermediate level of information processing – comprising the underlying assumptions (UAs) or conditional beliefs.

Two other chapters in this book are focused on identifying and restructuring negative core beliefs (CBs) and schemas, conceptualized as the third and deeper level of information processing (Wenzel, 2012; de-Oliveira, 2012).

2. Cognitive model

Cognitions may be assessed on at least three levels (Fig. 1). On a more superficial level of information processing, cognitions are known as ATs. Hollon & Kendall (1980) developed the Automatic Thoughts Questionnaire (ATQ-30), a 30-item questionnaire conceived to measure the frequency of occurrence of ATs, typically expressed as negative self-statements, and associated with depression. In the intermediate level of information processing, cognitions are usually called UAs or conditional beliefs. Weissman & Beck (1978) developed the Dysfunctional Attitude Scale to assess negative attitudes of depressed patients towards self, the outside world, and the future. Finally, in the deepest level of information processing, cognitions are known as CBs or schemas. Beck et al. (2001) proposed the Personality Beliefs Questionnaire, and Young and Brown (1994) developed the Young Schema Questionnaire to assess these beliefs.

It is largely recognized that cognitions and their relation to emotional and behavioral responses are complex phenomena. Fig. 1 illustrates the highly complex interactions between different elements of the cognitive model and the reciprocal influences of each element over the others.

Cognitive model

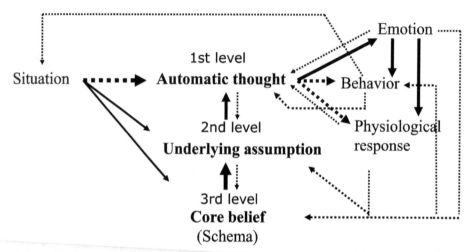

Fig. 1. Complex interactions between cognitions and responses to cognitions. (Copyright: Irismar Reis de Oliveira; http://trial-basedcognitivetherapy.com)

The full arrows seen in Fig. 1 represent more direct effects and the interrupted arrows represent possible indirect effects in the chain of elements triggered by a situation. This is important, for instance, when the therapist explains why different situations provoke different reactions (interrupted arrow between *situation* and *AT*) in different people or in the same people in different situations. Considering this complex model, a diagram that could make these interactions more easily understandable for the client during the therapeutic process would be particularly useful.

3. Case conceptualization

Case conceptualization is a key element in cognitive-behavioral therapy (CBT), and may be defined as a description of a patient's presenting problems that uses theory to make explanatory inferences about causes and maintaining factors, as well as to inform interventions (Kuyken et al, 2005). However, sharing its components with patients may be a complex and difficult task. As a highly individualized work, it should be collaboratively built with the client, while educating him/her about the cognitive model. While there are numerous case conceptualization diagrams proposed by different authors for different disorders and problems, Judith Beck's diagram is the most well known and used (J.S. Beck, 1995).

I designed a conceptualization diagram (shown in Figs. 2 and 3) to make the cognitive model easier to be understood by the client during therapy. It was developed for use in

Trial-Based Cognitive Therapy (de-Oliveira, 2011), but not limited to this approach, as its components are the same ones found in conventional CBT.

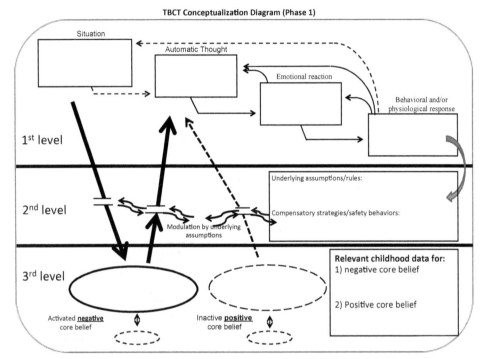

Fig. 2. TBCT conceptualization diagram showing an activated negative core belief. (Copyright: Irismar Reis de Oliveira; http://trial-basedcognitivetherapy.com)

In the first level of information processing shown in Fig. 2, a situation appraised by the patient as dangerous (*AT* box) would elicit anxiety (*emotional reaction* box) that could paralyze him/her (*behavioral and physiological responses* box). Arrows returning to the *emotional reaction*, *ATs* and *situation* boxes inform the patient about the circular nature of these interactions (confirmatory bias) that prevent him/her from reappraising the situation and consequently changing the erroneous perceptions it triggered.

This diagram might also be useful to make the patient understand that behaviors used in specific situations that elicit less anxiety and consequently yield a sense of immediate relief (e.g., avoidance) may progressively become a *safety behavior* (arrow directed from the *behavioral and physiological responses* box from the first to the second level on the right side of the picture). This means that perceptions in the first level may progressively become *UAs* or *rules* that are now maintained by the *compensatory strategies* and *safety behaviors* (confirmatory bias) seen in the second level. Safety behaviors then assume a modulatory function. Under the influence of the UAs that support such behaviors, first level appraisals (ATs) may be repeatedly confirmed. Also, third level (unconditional) *CBs* may be activated if UAs are challenged (for example, during exposure), or inactivated if UAs are not challenged (for example, by avoidance).

Having sufficient practice in identifying and changing ATs by replacing them with more functional alternative appraisals, the patient may progressively notice changes in the other levels, for instance, activation of positive CBs. However, restructuring negative CBs (see chapters 2 and 3 in this book.) is considered an important step for more durable results in therapy. Fig. 3 graphically illustrates such changes.

4. Dysfunctional ATs and cognitive distortions

ATs are rapid, evaluative thoughts that do not arise from deliberation or reasoning; as a result, the person is likely to accept them as true, without analysis (J.S. Beck, 1995). It is not uncommon for ATs to be distorted, and result in dysfunctional emotional reactions and behaviors that, in turn, produce more cognitive errors that maintain the vicious circle (level 1 of Fig. 1).

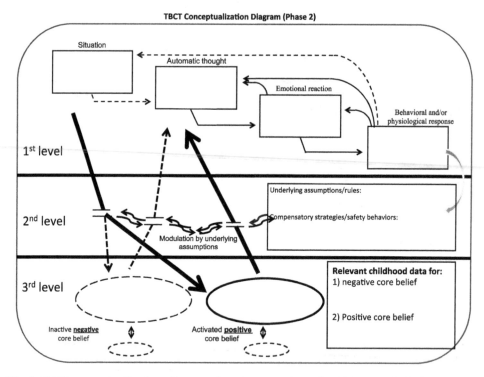

Fig. 3. TBCT conceptualization diagram showing an activated positive core belief. (Copyright: Irismar Reis de Oliveira; http://trial-basedcognitivetherapy.com).

Table 1 includes 15 known cognitive distortions, their definitions and examples (Burns, 1980; Beck, 1976; J.S. Beck 1995; Dryden & Ellis, 2001; Leahy, 2003). Teaching the patient to identify cognitive distortions is an important step to restructure such dysfunctional ATs. This may be done by means of the Intrapersonal Thought Record (IntraTR) described below. It is illustrated with the case of a panic disorder patient.

	Cognitive distortions	Definitions	Examples
1	Dichotomous thinking (also called all-or-nothing, black and white, or polarized thinking)	I view a situation, a person or an event only in all-or-nothing terms, fitting them into only two extreme categories instead of on a continuum.	"I made a mistake, therefore I'm a failure". "I ate more than I planned, so I blew my diet completely" **My example:**
2	Fortune telling (also called catastrophizing)	I predict the future in negative terms and believe that what will happen will be so awful that I will not be able to stand it	"I will fail and this will be unbearable." "I'll be so upset that I won't be able to concentrate for the exam." **My example:**
3	Discounting or disqualifying the positive	I disqualify and discount positive experiences or events insisting that they do not count."	"I passed the exam, but I was just lucky." "Going to college is not a big deal, anyone can do it." **My example:**
4	Emotional reasoning	I believe my emotions reflect reality and let them guide my attitudes and judgments.	"I feel she loves me, so it must be true." "I am terrified of airplanes, so flying must be dangerous." **My example:**
5	Labeling	I put a fixed, global label, usually negative, on myself or others.	"I'm a loser." "He's a rotten person." "She's a complete jerk." **My example:**
6	Magnification/minimization	I evaluate myself, others, and situations magnifying the negatives and/or minimizing the positives.	"I got a B. This proves how inferior I am." "I got an A. It doesn't mean I'm smart." **My example:**
7	Selective abstraction (also called mental filter and tunnel vision)	I pay attention to one or a few details and fail to see the whole picture	"My boss said he liked my presentation, but since he corrected a slide, I know he did not mean it." "Even though the group said my work was good, one person pointed out an error so I know I will be fired." **My example:**
8	Mind reading	I believe that I know the thoughts or intentions of others (or that they know my thoughts or intentions) without having sufficient evidence.	"He's thinking that I failed". "She thought I didn't know the project." "He knows I do not like to be touched this way." **My example:**
9	Overgeneralization	I take isolated cases and generalize them widely by means of words such as "always", "never", "everyone", etc.	"Every time I have a day off from work, it rains." "You only pay attention to me when you want sex". **My example:**

10	Personalizing	I assume that others' behaviors and external events concern (or are directed to) myself without considering other plausible explanations.	"I felt disrespected because the cashier did not say thank you to me" (not considering that the cashier did not say thank you to anyone). "My husband left me because I was a bad wife"(not considering that she was his fourth wife). **My example:**
11	Should statements (also "musts", "oughts", "have tos")	I tell myself that events, people's behaviors, and my own attitudes "should" be the way I expected them to be and not as they really are.	"I should have been a better mother". "He should have married Ann instead of Mary". "I shouldn't have made so many mistakes." **My example:**
12	Jumping to conclusions	I draw conclusions (negative or positive) from little or no confirmatory evidence.	"As soon as I saw him I knew he had bad intentions." "He was looking at me, so I concluded immediately he thought I was responsible for the accident". **My example:**
13	Blaming (others or oneself)	I direct my attention to others as sources of my negative feelings and experiences, failing to consider my own responsibility; or, conversely, I take responsibility for others' behaviors and attitudes.	'My parents are the ones to blame for my unhappiness." "It is my fault that my son married a selfish and uncaring person." **My example:**
14	What if?	I keep asking myself questions such as "what if something happens?"	"What if my car crashes?" "What if I have a heart attack?" "What if my husband leaves me?" **My example:**
15	Unfair comparisons	I compare myself with others who seem to do better than I do and place myself in a disadvantageous position.	"My father always preferred my elder brother because he is much smarter than I am." "I am a failure because she is more successful than I am." **My example:**

Table 1. Cognitive distortions, definitions and examples. (Copyright: Irismar Reis de Oliveira; http://trial-basedcognitivetherapy.com).

4.1 Intrapersonal thought record

A premise of CBT is that exaggerated or biased cognitions often maintain or exacerbate stressful states such as depression, anxiety, and anger (Leahy, 2003).

Beck et al. (1979) developed the Dysfunctional Thought Record (DTR) as a worksheet to help patients respond to ATs more effectively, thereby modifying negative mood states. This approach is useful for many patients who use the DTR consistently. However, for some patients, the alternative thoughts generated through the DTR and intended to be perceived as adaptive and rational may still lack credibility (de-Oliveira, 2008). To address this issue, Greenberger & Padesky (1995) expanded the original 5-column DTR designed by Beck et al. (1979) to seven columns. The two additional columns were evidence columns, allowing the patient to include evidence that does and does not support the ATs, enabling the patient to develop more balanced thoughts, and thus improve associated emotional reactions and behaviors.

I devised the IntraTR in order to make the restructuring of ATs easier for the patient, and to allow him/her to connect the ATs to the conceptualization diagram shown in Figs. 2 and 3. The following case vignette of a panic disorder patient illustrates how the IntraTR and the conceptualization diagram can be used together in order to restructure dysfunctional ATs (de-Oliveira, 2011b).

4.1.1 Case illustration

Sean, aged 35, had a 10-year history of frequent panic attacks with increasingly severe agoraphobia. SSRIs and benzodiazepines reduced his panic attacks' intensity and frequency, but his agoraphobia worsened, and for 3 years Sean had rarely left home alone. His fear of travelling even when accompanied limited his professional and personal life (his fiancée lived 200 miles away). Sean had 10 treatment sessions over 3 months. In session 1, he learned that fear and anxiety were normal, was introduced to the cognitive model (level 1 of the conceptualization diagram), and did interoceptive exposure by hyperventilating.

Sean was asked to learn about the cognitive distortions as homework. He received from the therapist a sheet (Table 1) containing names (column 1), definitions (column 2) and examples (column 3) of cognitive distortions. Also, Sean was asked to write down his own examples of cognitive distortions during the week in the space identified as "My example" in column 3 of Table 1. Identifying his own examples prepared Sean to be introduced to the Cognitive Distortions Questionnaire (CD-Quest) and the IntraTR, to be explored in session 2. In session 2, Sean completed the CD-Quest and an IntraTR in order to restructure his catastrophic ATs (e.g. "I'll lose control and go mad"). In session 3, Sean filled in 2 more IntraTRs. The CD-Quest was filled in weekly during the whole therapy process.

Fig. 4 illustrates Sean's conceptualization diagram, and Fig. 5 is the IntraTR filled in by Sean in session 2. In a situation in which he was preparing himself to go to work, he noticed his heart racing (situation box). Sean had the AT "I will have an attack again" (AT box), and felt anxious (emotional reaction box). Consequently, Sean decided not to go to work (behavioral and physiological response box). The therapist asked Sean to examine the cognitive distortions sheet (Table 1) in order to identify possible thinking errors and fill in item 1 of the IntraTR (Fig. 5). Sean came up with fortune telling and catastrophizing. Items 2 and 3 of the IntraTR helped Sean to uncover the evidence supporting and not supporting the AT. Sean was then asked to find out any advantages of behaving according to the AT (item 4). The answer was "No, because it makes me feel vulnerable." The therapist asked Sean how he could test the credibility of the AT (item 5) and the answer was: "Expose myself more." Sean was then stimulated to bring an alternative, more adaptive, hypothesis to replace the AT, one which could better explain the situation. Sean said: "This is just my heart racing. My amygdala is again hyperactive," was considered a more plausible and credible explanation, which he believed 70%. His anxiety fell to 40%, and he became able to go to work. After this work, Sean believed the AT (item 7) only 30%, and felt much better (item 8).[*]

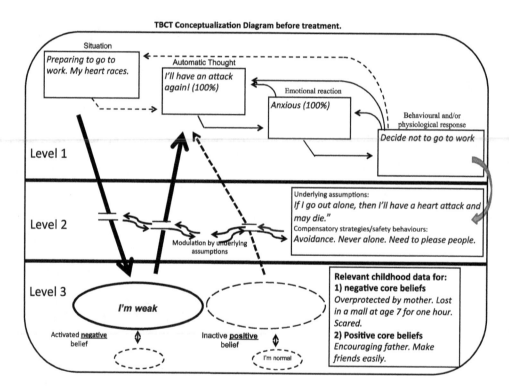

Fig. 4. Sean's TBCT conceptualization diagram filled in at the beginning of treatment. (Copyright: Irismar Reis de Oliveira; http://trial-basedcognitivetherapy.com).

---

[*]Sean's complete treatment may be assessed in the Common Language for Psychotherapy (CLP) procedures website (Trial-based cognitive therapy: http://www.commonlanguagepsychotherapy.org).

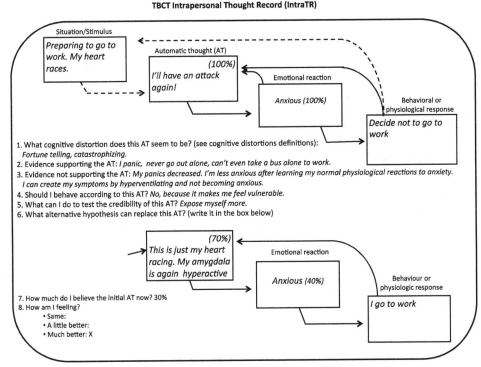

Fig. 5. One of Sean's IntraTRs filled in at the beginning of treatment (Copyright: Irismar Reis de Oliveira; http://trial-basedcognitivetherapy.com).

4.2 CD-Quest

The Cognitive Distortions Questionnaire (CD-Quest) was developed as an operational instrument, to be routinely used by patients to facilitate perceptions of the link between cognitive errors and their consequent emotional states, as well as dysfunctional behaviors (de-Oliveira et al. 2011). Also, it was designed to help therapists quantitatively assess and follow the clinical evolution of patients by means of its scores. It comprises 15 items that assess known cognitive distortions in two dimensions. The scores may range from 0 to 75.

In the first study conducted by our group (de-Oliveira et al. 2011), the initial psychometric properties of the CD-Quest in its Brazilian Portuguese version in a sample of university students were assessed. Medical and psychology students (n = 184; age = 21.8 ± 3.37) were evaluated using the following instruments: CD-Quest, Beck Depression Inventory (BDI), Beck Anxiety Inventory (BAI), and the Automatic Thoughts Questionnaire (ATQ). These self-report instruments were applied collectively in classrooms. The CD-Quest showed good internal consistency (0.83 - 0.86) and concurrent validity with BDI (0.65), BAI (0.51), and ATQ (0.65). Furthermore, it was able to discriminate between groups possessing depressive (BDI ≥ 12) and anxious (BAI ≥ 11) indicators from those not possessing such indicators (p < .001). An exploratory factor analysis by means of principal components analysis with varimax rotation showed the presence of four factors that together explained 56.6% of data variance. The factors consisted of the following types of cognitive distortions: (a) Factor I: dichotomous thinking, selective abstraction, personalizing, should statements, what if..., unfair comparisons; (b) Factor II: emotional reasoning, labeling, mind reading, jumping to conclusions; (c) Factor III: fortune telling, discounting positives, magnification / minimization; and (d) Factor IV: overgeneralizing, blaming. It was concluded that the CD-Quest was characterized by good psychometric properties, justifying the need for larger studies designed to determine its predictive validity, expand its construct validity, and measure the degree to which it is a useful measure of change achieved by patients in cognitive behavioral therapy.

5. UAs and safety behaviors

Behavioral experiments are amongst the most powerful strategies for bringing about change in CBT (Bennett-Levy et al. 2004), and provide a meeting ground for communication between knowledge derived from the rational mind and emotional mind (Padesky, 2004). Behavioral experiments are especially used to change UAs. These cognitions are expressed as conditional beliefs such as "If I go out alone, then I will have a heart attack and may die." Consequently, he or she usually avoids feared situations. In session 4 (see case illustration above), Sean was helped to go over his conceptualization diagram (Fig. 4), and understand that exposing himself to feared situations (for example, going out alone to work) was necessary to overcome unpleasant emotions and behaviors. Consensual Role-Play (CRP), a 7-step decision-making method, was proposed by the therapist to facilitate Sean's behavioral experiments (e.g. go out alone), and to challenge his safety behaviors (e.g. avoidance).

Fig. 6 shows how therapist and patients can increase the chance of the patient confronting situations made difficult by UAs and repeatedly reinforced safety behaviors. For example, Sean was encouraged to list advantages and disadvantages of coming alone to the therapy session (step 1). Then, he was helped by the therapist to confront the dissonance between "reason" and "emotion" (Padesky, 2004). For instance, Sean gave a 70% weight to advantages of going out alone (versus 30% for disadvantages) according to reason, but 90% weight to disadvantages of going out alone (versus 10% for advantages) according to emotion (step 2). By means of the empty chair approach (Greenberg, 2011), the therapist asked Sean to reach a consensus between "reason" and "emotion" in a 15-minute dialogue (step 3). After this step, the therapist asked Sean to assess the weight of advantages vs. disadvantages, coming to a consensus between rational and emotional perspectives. Sean was able to give an 80% weight for the advantages of going out alone vs. 20% weight for the disadvantages of going out alone (step 4). Next, after a debriefing of what Sean learned from this analysis (step 5), the therapist asked him if he was ready to make a decision: the answer was "yes," and Sean decided that he was able to try going out alone as an experiment (step 6). In order to increase the chances of success, the therapist helped Sean organize an action plan (Greenberger & Padesky, 1995), so that not only could Sean organize what to do, but he could also anticipate obstacles and find their solutions (step 7).

Another strategy that may help patients to increase the chances of doing behavioral experiments is providing a hierarchy of symptoms to which they are supposed to be exposed in order to obtain symptom remission. After collecting a detailed list of symptoms (e.g., OCD or social phobia symptoms), in which the patient scores each one according to the hierarchy shown in Fig. 7, the therapist informs him/her that there will be no focus on blue symptoms, but he/she will choose 2 or 3 green symptoms to practice exposure as homework during the week. In general, the therapist uses CRP to help patients accept to expose themselves to yellow symptoms, usually during therapy sessions. These are symptoms patients resist to confront when they are alone, and CRP seems to make this challenge acceptable, at least in the therapist's presence. The therapist explains to the patient that he/she will NEVER need to challenge red symptoms. This information tends to make the patient more willing to comply with the technique because there is no pressure to confront the most anxiety provoking items. Therapist and patient keep track of individual and global symptom scores weekly. The patients notice that the scores continue to decrease (both those which he/she exposed him/herself to and those which he/she did not expose him/herself to). Patients are very surprised to realize that even red symptoms scores decrease, making exposure acceptable because they gradually become yellow or green. Showing the patient a global score chart helps him/her track weekly progress and notice scores change. The symptoms list to be filled out weekly is presented to the patient in a way that past scores are hidden, so that he/she will not be influenced by past symptoms scores.

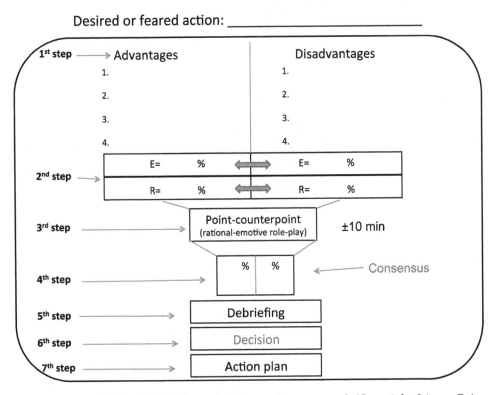

Fig. 6. Consensual role-play (CRP) as a decision-making approach (Copyright: Irismar Reis de Oliveira; http://trial-basedcognitivetherapy.com).

Patient's name: ....

Please, choose the scores (0-5) corresponding to what you would feel if you were to expose yourself to each item below.

Session	01	02	03	04	05	06	07	08	09	10	11	12	13	14	15	16	17	18	19	20
Date	/	/	/	/	/	/	/	/	/	/	/	/	/	/	/	/	/	/	/	/
Go to the supermarket	5	5	5	5	5	5	4													
Go out	5	4	3	3	3	1	0													
Touch objects coming from street	5	5	5	5	4	3	3													
Touch people	5	5	5	5	5	5	4													
Be touched by people	5	5	5	5	5	5	4													
Touch money	5	5	5	5	5	5	5													
Eat with hands	4	4	3	2	1	0	0													
Not washing hands	5	5	5	5	5	4	2													
Touch telephone	5	5	5	5	5	5	4													
Touch door knob	5	5	5	5	5	5	5													
Not discard towel after bath	3	2	1	0	0	0	0													
Work with computer	2	2	2	1	0	0	0													
Touch mail	3	3	3	2	2	1	0													
Touch shoes	5	5	5	5	5	5	5													
Touch/hug daughters	5	5	4	4	3	2	0													
Kiss daughters	5	5	4	3	3	3	0													
Kiss and being kissed by others	5	5	5	5	4	4	3													
Wash dishes	2	1	0	0	0	0	0													
Touch my string of beads	1	0	0	0	0	0	0													
Touch therapist's hand	2	1	0	0	0	0	0													
Touch my books	3	3	3	2	1	0	0													
TOTAL SCORE (sum of individual items)	85	80	73	67	61	53	39													
Number of exposures you do not allow yourself to do (reds and yellows)	14	14	12	11	10	9	7													

Table 2. Scores of OCD symptoms according to the Color Coded Symptom Hierarchy card in a patient.

0 =	Exposure is confortable or indifferent.
1 =	Exposure is slightly uncomfortable.
2 =	Exposure is clearly uncomfortable.
3 =	Exposure is very uncomfortable.
4 =	Exposure is so distressful that I do it only if really necessary.
5 =	Exposure is so distressful that I cannot imagine myself doing it.

Fig. 7. Color coded symptoms hierarchy card to facilitate exposure implementation
(Copyright: Irismar Reis de Oliveira; http://trial-basedcognitivetherapy.com).

6. Conclusion

Restructuring dysfunctional ATs is an important step in changing such superficial, but not least important, cognitions. However, because ATs are determined by the activation of negative core beliefs, restructuring and changing these beliefs is the most significant step for the patient. These procedures are shown in chapters 2 (Wenzel, 2012) and 3 (de-Oliveira, 2012) in this book. The present chapter illustrates how to introduce the cognitive model to the patients by means of a conceptualization diagram, using the IntraTR to help patients change ATs, and the CD-Quest to assess and challenge cognitive distortions. Finally, I introduced the CRP, and the color coded symptoms hierarchy card, strategies shaped to help patients make decisions involving the confrontation of safety behaviors, and consequently facilitating the modification of dysfunctional UAs.

7. References

[1] Alford BA, Beck AT (1997) The integrative power of cognitive therapy. Guilford, New York.
[2] Beck AT (1976) Cognitive therapy and the emotional disorders. International Universities Press, New York.
[3] Beck AT, Rush AJ, Shaw BF, Emery G (1979) Cognitive therapy of depression. Guilford Press, New York.
[4] Beck AT, Butler AC, Brown GK, Dahlsgaard KK, Newman CF, Beck JS (2001) Dysfunctional beliefs discriminate personality disorders. Behavioural Research Therapy, 39:1213-1225.
[5] Beck JS (1995) Cognitive therapy: basics and beyond. New York: Guilford Press.
[6] Bennett-Levy J (2004) Behavioural experiments: historical and conceptual underpinnings. In: Bennett-Levy J, Butler G, Fennel M, Hackmann A, Mueller M, Westrook D (eds) Oxford guide to behavioural experiments in cognitive therapy. Oxford, New York.
[7] Burns DD (1980) Feeling Good: The New Mood Therapy. New York: Signet.
[8] De-Oliveira IR (2008) Trial-Based Thought Record (TBTR): preliminary data on a strategy to deal with core beliefs by combining sentence reversion and the use of analogy with a judicial process. Jornal Brasileiro de Psiquiatria, 30:12-18.

[9] De-Oliveira IR (2011) Trial-based cognitive therapy: Accepted entry in Common Language for Psychotherapy Procedures (www.commonlanguagepsychotherapy.org, retrieved in August 7, 2011).

[10] De-Oliveira (2012) Use of the trial-based thought record to change dysfunctional core beliefs In: de-Oliveira IR (ed.) Cognitive-behavioral therapy. InTech, Rijeka, Croatia.

[11] De-Oliveira IR, Osório FL, Sudak D, Abreu JN, Crippa JAS, Powell VB, Landeiro F, Wenzel A (2011) Initial psychometric properties of the Cognitive Distortions Questionnaire (CD-Quest). Presented at the 45th Annual Meeting of the Association for Behavioral and Cognitive Therapies (ABCT), Toronto, Canada, November, 10-13.

[12] Dryden W, Ellis A (2001) Rational Emotive Behavior Therapy. In: Dobson KS, Handbook of Cognitive Behavioral Therapies. Guilford Press, New York.

[13] Greenberg LS (2011) Two-chair technique. Accepted entry in Common Language for Psychotherapy Procedures (www.commonlanguagepsychotherapy.org, retrieved in August 28, 2011).

[14] Greenberger D, Padesky CA (1995) Mind over mood. New York: Guilford Press.

[15] Hollon SD, Kendall PC (1980) Cognitive self-statements in depression: development of an automatic thoughts questionnaire. Cognitive Therapy and Research, 4:383-395.

[16] Kuyken W, Fothergill CD, Musa M, Chadwick P (2005) the reliability and quality of cognitive case formulation. Behaviour Research and Therapy, 43:1187-1201.

[17] Leahy RL (2003) Cognitive therapy techniques. A practitioner's guide. New York: Guilford Press.

[18] Padesky C (2004) Behavioural experiments: at the crossroads. In: Bennett-Levy J, Butler G, Fennel M, Hackmann A, Mueller M, and Westrook D (eds) Oxford guide to behavioural experiments in cognitive therapy. Oxford, New York.

[19] Weissman AN, Beck AT (1978) Development and validation of the Dysfunctional Attitude Scale: a preliminary investigation. Presented at the 62nd Annual Meeting of the American Educational Research Association, Toronto, Canada, March 27-31).

[20] Wenzel A (2011) Modification of Core Beliefs in Cognitive Therapy. In: de-Oliveira IR (ed.) Cognitive-behavioral therapy. InTech, Rijeka, Croatia.

[21] Young JE, Brown G (1994) Schema Questionnaire. In: Young JE (Ed.) Cognitive therapy for personality disorders: a schema focused approach. Sarasota, FL, Professional Resource Exchange.

3

Modification of Core Beliefs in Cognitive Therapy

Amy Wenzel

Wenzel Consulting, LLC,
Department of Psychiatry, University of Pennsylvania,
USA

1. Introduction

As has been seen in this volume thus far, a great deal of work in cognitive therapy is geared toward the identification, evaluation, and modification of situational thoughts (i.e., *automatic thoughts*) that patients experience on particular occasions and that are associated with an increase in an aversive mood state. Although they usually obtain significant relief from their mood disturbance using this *cognitive restructuring* process, many patients who focus only on these situational cognitions find that they continue to experience the same thoughts, over and over again, even if they have increased their ability to cope with them. One explanation for this is that these patients continue to hold unhelpful core beliefs, which facilitate the activation of these situational thoughts.

Core beliefs are defined as fundamental, inflexible, absolute, and generalized beliefs that people hold about themselves, others, the world, and/or the future (J. S. Beck, 2011; K. S. Dobson, 2012). When a core belief is inaccurate, unhelpful, and/or judgmental (e.g., "I am worthless"), it has a profound effect on a person's self-concept, sense of self-efficacy, and continued vulnerability to mood disturbance. Core beliefs typically center around themes of lovability (e.g., "I am undesirable"), adequacy ("I am incompetent"), and/or helplessness (e.g., "I am trapped"). I propose that the greatest amount of change, and the best prevention against relapse, results when patients identify unhelpful core beliefs and work with their therapists, using cognitive therapy strategies, to develop and embrace a healthier belief system.

Core beliefs are much more difficult to elicit and modify in cognitive therapy sessions, relative to situational automatic thoughts. They usually develop from messages received, over time, during a person's formative years, oftentimes during childhood but sometimes during times of substantial stress during adulthood. For example, consider the case of a female patient, "Cori," who was told repeatedly by her parents during childhood that she was worthless because the pregnancy was unwanted, her parents only married one another because it was the "right thing to do" once the pregnancy was discovered, and they viewed themselves as miserable ever since then. Not surprisingly, this woman was characterized by the core belief, "I'm worthless." Other patients receive messages from their peers that they are unwanted when they are teased and bullied. There are still other patients who had adaptive, healthy belief systems develop during childhood and adolescence, only to experience horrific events as an adult that had a profound impact on their core beliefs (e.g., a young man who joins the military and engages in combat returns home with the belief, "The world is cruel"). Identification of the pathway by which core beliefs develop can provide multiple points for intervention and evaluation.

It is important to understand the core belief construct's place in light of cognitive theory, as this knowledge will allow clinicians to understand and articulate to their patients the mechanism of change by which they expect therapeutic work on core beliefs to exert its desired effect. Figure 1 displays the central cognitive constructs in cognitive theory. The core belief construct is embedded in the larger construct of the *schema*. According to Clark and Beck (1999), schemas are "relatively enduring internal structures of stored generic or prototypical features of stimuli, ideas, or experience that are used to organize new information in a meaningful way thereby determining how phenomena are perceived and conceptualized" (p. 79). In other words, schemas not only influence *what* we believe (i.e., cognitive contents), but also *how* we process information that we encounter in our daily lives (i.e., information processing). Core beliefs, then, are the cognitive contents that are indicative of a person's schema. When a schema and its corresponding core belief(s) are activated, people process information in a biased manner, such that they attend to, assign importance to, encode, and retrieve information that is consistent with the schema, and they overlook information that is inconsistent with the schema. Thus, there is a bidirectional relation between information processing biases and core beliefs, such that information biases strengthen a person's core beliefs, and that core beliefs strengthen information processing biases. It is not difficult to imagine, for example, that a person with an unhelpful schema characterized by depressogenic core beliefs (e.g., "I'm a failure") will attend to information that reinforces those beliefs at the expense of neutral or contrary evidence, entrenching that person further in his or her depression.

Schemas and their corresponding core beliefs give rise to what Judith Beck has termed *intermediate beliefs* (J. S. Beck, 2011), which are defined as conditional rules, attitudes, and assumptions, often unspoken, that play a large role in the manner in which people live their lives and respond to life's challenges and stressors. In many instances, they are worded as "if-then" conditional statements that prescribe certain rules that must be met in order for the person to protect him- or herself from a painful core belief. For example, a person with an "I'm a failure" core belief might live by the rule, "If I get all As, then I'm successful," which is viewed as a positive intermediate belief because it specifies a path toward a positive outcome. However, that same person might also live by a negative intermediate belief, "If I get anything less than all As, then I'm a failure." Intermediate beliefs that do not use conditional language are often expressed as heavily valenced attitudes (e.g., "It would be terrible to get anything less than an A.") or assumptions about the way the world works (e.g., "Successful people should get all As in their classes."). The problem with these rules and assumptions is that they are rigid and inflexible, usually prescribing impossible standards to which one should live his or her life and failing to account for life's unexpected events and challenges that invariably affect one's ability to achieve these standards. As with core beliefs, they exacerbate information processing biases that reinforce unhelpful core beliefs, and conversely, information processing biases strengthen the rigidity of these rules and assumptions.

It is not surprising, then, that schemas and their associated core beliefs, intermediate beliefs, and information processing biases create a context for certain automatic thoughts to arise under particular circumstances. Continuing with the example in the previous paragraph, if a person is characterized by a failure core belief and carries rigid rules about the meaning of grades he receives in school, then receiving a "D" on a test might be associated with the automatic thoughts, "I'm never going to get into medical school; My life will be meaningless." However, consider another person who has the core belief "I'm unlovable" and who carries rigid rules about the meaning of her accomplishments on the degree to which others value her. In this case, receiving a "D" on a test might be associated with the automatic thoughts, "I have nothing to contribute to anyone; why should anyone care about me?" This comparative illustration demonstrates that two people in similar situations can report very different automatic thoughts, and the explanation for those different thought patterns is that these people are characterized by different sets of core beliefs and intermediate beliefs. Information processing biases only serve to further increase the likelihood that patients will experience negative automatic thoughts in stressful or otherwise challenging situations, and when the thoughts are activated, they feed back into those biases.

A final cognitive construct in this model is that of the mode, captured in the upper right-hand corner of Figure 1. According to A. T. Beck (1996), a *mode* is an interrelated set of schemas. Thus, several systems of schemas, core beliefs, intermediate beliefs, automatic thoughts, and information processing biases can be assimilated into a larger mode. A. T. Beck proposed three types of modes: (a) those that are primal in nature, which influence basic and immediate necessities such as preservation and security; (b) those that are constructive in nature, which influence the ability to have effective relationships and build life satisfaction; and (c) those that are minor in nature, which influence daily activities such as reading, writing and driving. As anyone who has treated a psychiatric patient has undoubtedly seen, unhelpful belief systems have the potential to severely limit patients' functioning in all three of these modal domains.

I propose that core beliefs play a central role in cognitive theory and that modification of core beliefs will play a fundamental role in modifying the other layers of cognition in the cognitive model. The adoption of a healthy belief system is hypothesized to add flexibility and even a sense of kindness to patients' rules and assumptions by which they live their lives, which is proposed to, in turn, decrease the likelihood that unhelpful situational thoughts will be activated automatically in stressful or challenging situations. A healthy belief system might to decrease the weight that unhelpful schemas carry when people function in various modes. I also hypothesize that the adoption of a healthy belief system will decrease the extremity of unhelpful information processing biases, as patients will begin to widen the scope of the information to which they attend to and process in their environment. I acknowledge that other cognitive behavioral approaches to treatment focus primarily on the modification of other constructs in this model, such as Nader Amir's attentional modification program that uses a computer task to train patients' attention away from stimuli that reinforces their pathology (Amir, Beard, Burns, & Bomyea, 2009; Amir, Beard, Taylor, et al., 2009). Nevertheless, I believe that an intentional focus on core beliefs during the course of cognitive therapy has the greatest potential to help patients create a healthy belief system, which will in turn increase functioning in many domains of their lives.

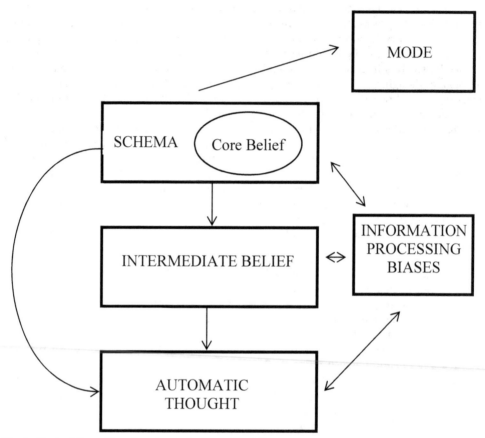

Fig. 1. Central Cognitive Constructs in Cognitive Theory.

In this chapter, I describe strategies for identifying and modifying unhelpful core beliefs. Throughout this chapter, I illustrate the application of these strategies with cases that I have seen or supervised in my practice, taking care to remove and modify any identifying information. I conclude the chapter with a discussion of challenges that can arise when working with core beliefs and directions for future research.

2. Identification of core beliefs

The first step in working with patients' core beliefs is for the therapist and patient to, collaboratively, identify them. Some patients present in the first session with a clear understanding of their core beliefs; for example, a patient, "Karen," articulated in her first session that the main issue she wanted to address was her belief that she is inferior to those whom she perceives as more accomplished than her. It is more common, however, for patients to need some time before they can identify and are ready to work with core beliefs. For example, some patients have difficulty identifying the cognitions that are related to aversive mood states, so they require practice with the more-easily-accessible automatic thoughts before they have a sense of their underlying core beliefs. Other patients, early in therapy, find articulation of their core beliefs to be overly threatening and painful, and working with situational automatic thoughts allows them to develop a comfort level in working with their cognitions before they begin to focus on their most fundamental beliefs (K. S. Dobson, 2012). For these reasons, most cognitive therapists work with situational automatic thoughts earlier in the course of treatment and with core beliefs later in the course of treatment.

When therapists opt to work with patients across several sessions, focusing first on situational automatic thoughts, they can be vigilant for the presence of core beliefs through several means. For example, automatic thoughts that provoke a great deal of affect have the potential to be core beliefs in and of themselves, or be a direct manifestation of a core belief. Patients who systematically track their automatic thoughts across several sessions (e.g., through the use of Dysfunctional Thoughts Record) can begin to identify themes in the thoughts that they identify, which may provide a clue about the nature of the underlying core belief. When patients spontaneously report recurrent experiences that remind them of another experience, the therapist can take the opportunity to identify the threads that link these experiences together and the messages they internalized from them—both of which could reflect their core beliefs (D. Dobson & Dobson, 2009).

Perhaps the most commonly recognized strategy for identifying core beliefs is the *Downward Arrow Technique*, first mentioned by A. T. Beck, Rush, Shaw, and Emery (1979) and subsequently elaborated upon by Burns (1980). Therapists who use this strategy ask repeatedly about the meaning of situational automatic thoughts until they arrive upon a core belief, whose meaning is so fundamental that there is no additional meaning associated with it. Take, for instance, a socially anxious patient, "Gary," who was treated with 12 sessions of cognitive therapy. This patient's presenting concern was excessive blushing and blotchiness, for which he perceived that others would judge him negatively. In describing a social situation in which he was convinced that he was becoming red, he identified the automatic thought, "Others are going to see that I am red." Figure 2 displays the application of the downward arrow technique for this case. It is evident that this exercise elicited a pair of powerful core beliefs, "I am weak" and "I am less than a man."

Many therapists administer self-report inventories to assess identify cognitions that have the potential to be core beliefs. These questionnaires include: (a) the Dysfunctional Attitudes Scale (DAS; Weissman & Beck, 1980); (b) the Sociotropy-Autonomy Scale (SAS; Bieling, Beck, & Brown, 2000; D. A. Clark & Beck, 1991);(c) the Personality Belief Questionnaire (PBQ; A. T. Beck & Beck, 1991; A. T. Beck et al., 2001), and (d) the Young Schema Questionnaire (YSQ; http://www.schematherapy.com/id49.htm). Advantages of administering inventories of this nature are that core beliefs can be identified in a relatively short period of time and that an extensive range of possible beliefs can be considered. This allows the therapist to develop a richer case conceptualization than he or she might otherwise develop on the basis of interview and observational information alone. However, it is important to regard core beliefs identified via self-report inventories as hypotheses to be tested using the "data" that are obtained by the therapeutic work that takes place across sessions. As stated previously, early in the course of treatment, many patients are not aware of their core beliefs. This lack of awareness could influence the manner in which they respond to these inventories, such that they minimize the operation of one or more beliefs. Moreover, core beliefs are idiosyncratic to each individual, so there is always the possibility that a salient core belief is not assessed on the inventory that is administered. D. Dobson and Dobson (2009) have recommended that self-report inventories of core beliefs should be administered after patients' immediate distress has been addressed, so that their distress does not affect their responses to items on the inventory, but not so late in treatment that their beliefs have already shifted.

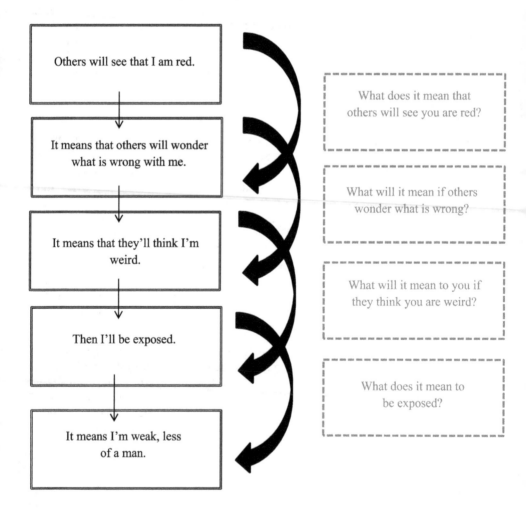

Fig. 2. Application of the Downward Arrow Technique.

3. Modification of core beliefs

Because they are so entrenched, core beliefs are almost never modified after only one session of cognitive therapy. More typically, once core beliefs are identified, the therapist and patient work together, collaboratively, to decrease the degree to which the patient believes the old, unhelpful core belief and increase the degree to which the patient believes a new, healthier belief. In this section, I describe some common strategies for the modification of core beliefs. Most therapists use a creative combination of the strategies described in this session (as well as other strategies) to achieve core belief modification with their patients.

3.1 Defining the core belief

In most cases, core beliefs are so global that they pervade all aspects of a patient's life (e.g., "I'm a failure," "I'm worthless."). However, patients take these excessive judgments as fact without taking the time to operationalize the components that comprise them. When patients are faced with identification of the components that make up successfulness, worth, lovability and so on, they often realize that they are basing their judgment on one or two areas of their lives that are not going well for them and failing to acknowledge the other areas of their lives that contribute to these constructs are going rather well. Thus, a first step I take in modifying core beliefs is to work with patients to define their components so that we know, more precisely, what is driving the belief, so that we can gain perspective on the belief, and so that we can identify specific points of intervention.

One straightforward way to define the components of core beliefs is to use a pie chart. Figure 3 displays a pie chart for a depressed and angry patient, "Marco," who had the core belief, "I'm not as good as others." He divided his pie into components that he believed contributed to a person's ability to, indeed, be as good as others. As can be seen in Figure 1, Marco put the greatest weight on his career, the second greatest amount of weight on a romantic relationship, the third greatest amount of weight on major possessions, and an equal amount of weight on relationships with his children and recreational pursuits. Notice that some of these components required definitions, themselves. For example, Marco was encouraged to identify the most important aspects of his career that would help him to adopt the new core belief, that he is as good as other people. He also identified the number of recreational pursuits that would reinforce this new core belief, as well as the types of possessions he would have that would, in his view, be manifestations of being as good as other people.

There may be aspects of the components of a patient's core belief that the therapist views as concerning. For example, it appears that Marco is one whose self-worth is driven, at least to some degree, by money, status, and possessions. Therapists must remember that it is not their place to judge patients' priorities and values, but rather to help them identify discrepancies between their current life situation and their beliefs, values, and aspirations. Regardless, defining the components of Marco's core belief in this manner allowed Marco and his therapist to examine his functioning in five different domains, evaluate the degree to which his view of his functioning in these five domains is accurate and helpful, and to identify action plans for improving functioning in these five domains.

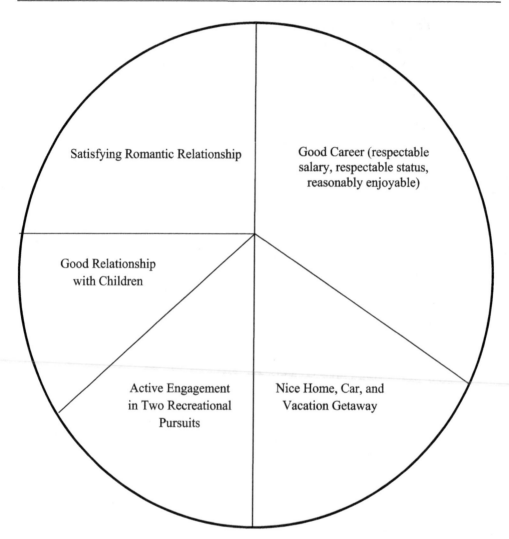

Fig. 3. Sample Pie Chart to Define "Being As Good As Others".

3.2 Examining evidence

A common strategy for modifying core beliefs is to critically examine the evidence that supports the old, unhelpful core belief and that which supports a new, healthier core belief. The goal is for, over time, the patient to accumulate an increasing amount of evidence that supports the new core belief, which in turn is expected to be associated with an increase in the degree to which the patient believes the new belief and a decrease in the degree to which the patient believes the old core belief. When the patient identifies evidence that supports the old core belief, the therapist works with the patient to use cognitive restructuring strategies to reframe it. Judith Beck (2011) has created a *Core Belief Worksheet* to achieve this goal. Other therapists do not use a formal worksheet, but instead have their patients keep track of this evidence over time on a *Positive Data Log* (D. Dobson & Dobson, 2009).

Recall the patient, Cori, introduced earlier in the chapter. She carried the core belief, "I'm worthless" throughout her adult life on the basis of consistent, negative messages that she received from her parents during childhood. Until she participated in cognitive therapy, she ignored positive feedback that she received from others, which could very well have implications for her belief of worthlessness. When she participated in cognitive therapy, she agreed to keep a Positive Data Log, writing down the feedback that she received from others that suggest that others see her as having a great deal of worth. After completing this exercise, she could not deny that others—her children, her co-workers, and people at church—valued her highly, and she concluded that she had some worth. Of course, it, ultimately, is important that Cori can view herself as having worth even without positive feedback from others. However, this exercise was the catalyst in putting a significant dent in her belief that she is worthless, allowing her and her therapist to develop creative strategies to help her, on her own, acknowledge that she has worth. Without the Positive Data Log, she would have rejected this notion.

Marco, on the other hand, drew a different conclusion after examining the evidence that contributed to his core belief that he is not as good as other people. He determined that he was not where he would like to be in all five areas that he believed contributed to being "good enough"—career, possessions, romantic relationship, relationship with his children, and consistent engagement in meaningful and enjoyable recreational activities. On the basis of this conclusion, he and his therapist used graded task assignment (Wenzel, Brown, & Karlin, 2011) to break each of these areas into smaller pieces and used problem solving to begin to make positive changes in his life, with the idea that each positive change will bring him closer to living his life consistent with the new, healthier core belief, "I'm as good as other people."

These case illustrations demonstrate that, although examination of the evidence that supports new, healthier core beliefs is a central activity that occurs in cognitive therapy, it is usually not a strategy that is an end in and of itself. Rather, it allows the patient and therapist to begin to modify the belief so that the patient is able to tolerate other creative therapeutic interventions that will solidify the shift in beliefs.

3.3 Advantages-disadvantages analysis

The *advantages-disadvantages analysis* is a versatile strategy that can be used for many purposes in cognitive therapy, such as evaluating potential solutions to problems or for weighing the pros and cons of decisions that patients face in their daily lives. It can also be used during core belief modification to help patients draw conclusions about the utility of their core beliefs after examining their advantages and disadvantages. To conduct the advantages-disadvantages analysis, patients draw a 4 X 4 quadrant, with the old core belief and the new core belief listed across the top, and "advantages" and "disadvantages" listed down the side. Then, patients record the advantages and disadvantages of each belief.

The advantages-disadvantages analysis can be used for a patient like Gary, who, after examining the evidence that supported and refuted the beliefs that he is weak and less than a man, still held onto his unhelpful beliefs. Specifically, he continued to believe that turning red and blotchy in social situations made him weak and less than a man, reasoning that other men did not have to deal with such a "flaw" and that he could not even do what other men take for granted. His therapist turned to the advantages-disadvantages analysis to examine the degree to which holding on to such beliefs were working for him or working against him. Figure 4 displays Gary's advantages-disadvantages analysis. After completing this exercise, Gary recognized that holding this core belief is likely to significantly increase the probability that he would, indeed, turn red and blotchy in social situations. He also concluded that it was keeping him from addressing more central issues in his life, such as a lack of fulfillment in his career.

	"I'm weak, I'm less than a man."	"I'm just as much of a man as other guys."
Advantages	• I keep working on overcoming my problems. • I protect myself from people seeing how red and blotchy I get.	• Maybe I would get less red and blotchy. • Maybe I would attend more social events and feel more relaxed. • I'd look more confident to women I want to date. • I would feel better about myself. • This problem would stop taking up so much time and energy. • I could move on and address some other areas of my life (e.g., getting my career on track).
Disadvantages	• When these beliefs are activated, I get even more anxious, red, and botchy. • They keep me from taking social risks (e.g., asking someone out on a date). • I avoid social activities that used to be a lot of fun. • When I do attend social events, I am preoccupied with whether I am turning red and blotchy. • I feel badly about myself. • They are keeping me from moving forward in my life (e.g., applying for a new job). • I'm not where I want to be in life.	• It seems hard to believe right now. • I could get red and blotchy, be rejected, and be devastated.

Fig. 4. Sample Advantages-Disadvantages Analysis.

As can be seen in this illustration, the advantages-disadvantages analysis usually provides a complex perspective on the core belief, as valid reasons for maintaining the unhelpful core belief are acknowledged. Unhelpful core beliefs can often be conceptualized as being understandable and associated with many advantages at the time they developed, but that, in the present, they are no longer associated with those advantages and now serve to exacerbate emotional distress. In addition, patients may view the adoption of new core beliefs as being associated with significant short-term disadvantages (e.g., discomfort), but also being associated with significant advantages in the long-term (D. Dobson & Dobson, 2009). In fact, K. S. Dobson (2012) has developed an expanded version of the advantages-disadvantages analysis, such that advantages and disadvantages of the old and new core beliefs are considered from short- and long-term time perspectives.

3.4 Behavioral experiments

Some patients find that they believe the results from strategies designed to modify core beliefs "intellectually" but that they still believe their old, unhelpful core belief "emotionally." In my experience, one explanation for this is that the verbal and written strategies described in the chapter to this point are not potent enough to provide a vivid demonstration that their core belief is inaccurate or unhelpful. *Behavioral experiments* are powerful experiential exercises that patients implement in their own lives, outside of session, to test aspects of core beliefs. In essence, a behavioral experiment requires the patient to formulate a prediction on the basis of a core belief and then gather "data" to support or refute that prediction. Patients "see for themselves" the degree to which their predictions and beliefs are warranted.

The implementation of a behavioral experiment is demonstrated with the patient described earlier in this chapter, Cori. Because she believes that she is worthless, Cori predicted that others would dismiss her contribution at her monthly book club meeting. In the past, she had refrained from sharing her comments and observations at these meetings, which further reinforced the belief that she is worthless because she believed she had nothing meaningful to share. To implement the behavioral experiment, Cori's therapist worked with her to (a) identify what she hoped to communicate about that month's book club selection, (b) practice articulating it, and (c) objectively observe others' reactions to her. At the subsequent session, Cori reported that there was no evidence that others rejected her contribution, and in fact, that two others in her book club noted that they had similar observations. Cori and her therapist discussed the manner in which her worthlessness core belief might be revised in light of this experience.

Many behavioral experiments involve, at least in part, an observation of others' reactions (e.g., the other members of Cori's book club). It is important for therapists to be mindful of the fact that they cannot control others' reactions and that there is a possibility that others will respond in a manner that inadvertently reinforces the patient's old, unhelpful core belief. Thus, behavioral experiments must be developed thoughtfully and thoroughly in session, in a manner that gives the patient an opportunity to have a "win-win" situation. In the previous example, Cori's therapist took the time to work with her on formulating the thoughts she hoped to share with the group and practicing effective communication skills. Cori's therapist also helped her to approach the experiment as if she were testing two competing predictions that contributed to her worthlessness belief. Cori predicted that other members of the book club would dismiss or reject her contribution, which, to her, was another indicator that she is worthless. Although Cori's therapist was confident of Cori's communication abilities and doubted that would occur, they also prepared for the worst case scenario (i.e., that the others would indeed dismiss or reject her contribution), which was associated with a related belief, "I'm so worthless that I can't cope with rejection." They developed specific coping skills for managing distress associated with a rebuff, and Cori's therapist framed Cori's use of these coping skills as evidence that she has worth because she is able to weather adversity.

3.5 Acting "as if"

At times, patients continue to engage in engrained and self-defeating behavioral patterns that reinforce their old, unhelpful core beliefs. *Acting "as if"* is a specific type of behavioral experiment in which patients behave in a manner consistent with a new, healthier belief (even if they are not fully invested in the new belief) and evaluate the effects of this new behavioral set. Questions patients can consider after acting "as if" include: (a) What were the effects on my mood (e.g., happier?, less anxious?); (b) How did others respond to me?, (c) What negative consequences came from my acting "as if"?; and (d) What positive consequences came from my acting "as if"? In most instances, patients see that acting according to a new, healthier belief frees them from their unhelpful core beliefs, allows them to let go of emotional distress, and elicits positive reactions from others.

Gary used acting "as if" to modify the belief that others would react negatively to him if he were to become red and botchy in a social situation, thereby exposing himself as being weak. When he first entered therapy, he presented with a submissive posture, not wanting anyone to notice him and comment on his appearance. His therapist hypothesized that this behavior actually increased the likelihood of negative reactions from others (e.g., by making others uncomfortable around him), thereby reinforcing his old, unhelpful core beliefs. His therapist encouraged Gary to act "as if" he did not care that he had a propensity to become red and blotchy and to carry himself with confidence. Gary implemented this assignment in the time in between sessions, and at his subsequent session, he reported that he had had dates with two different women that he had met at social engagements. As a result of this experiment, Gary began to see that he was overstating the implications of his propensity to turn red and blotchy and that, by carrying himself in a manner consistent with the core belief "I am just as much of a man as other guys," members of the opposite sex found him to be attractive and were interested in dating him.

3.6 Cognitive continuum

The *cognitive continuum* is a strategy for critically examining, and ultimately modifying, all-or-nothing core beliefs, such as "I'm a failure." Patients are asked to draw a horizontal line representing the full continuum of their core belief from 0% to 100%. For example, a patient with a core belief of "I'm a failure" might write the word "Failure" under the anchor for 0% and the word "Successful" under the anchor for 100%. The patient is asked to provide an initial rating of where on the continuum he or she falls, as well as the point on the continuum in which the negative core belief begins (e.g., failure begins at 20%). As the exercise progresses, the patient considers the full spectrum of people who would lie on the continuum and lists some of these people as anchors (e.g., people who would be considered at 10%, 20%, et cetera, through 80% and 90%). Concurrently, the patient continually revises where he or she stands on the basis of these anchors. In most instances, when patients consider the full spectrum of people who could be included on this continuum (which could range from world leaders to people who are in prison and homeless), they generally conclude that they compare favorably to many others and that they are doing no better or worse than most people.

It is important for therapists who use the cognitive continuum to be vigilant for distorted or inaccurate beliefs that fuel the location at which they place themselves on the continuum. Recall the patient, Karen, who was introduced earlier in the chapter. Karen was a physician's assistant and worried a great deal about being "found out" as incompetent, which contributed to her perception that she was inferior to others. Using the cognitive continuum, she initially rated herself as 30% on a continuum from competent (100%) to incompetent (0%) and estimated that incompetence started at 30%. She made her estimate on the basis of questionable reasoning; for example, she believed that she consulted her medical books much more frequently than other health care providers and interpreted that as a sign of incompetence. Thus, during the cognitive continuum exercise, Karen's therapist also worked with her to evaluate whether consulting her medical books was equal to being incompetent and whether there are other ways to view the consultation of her medical books (e.g., she cares deeply for her patients and wants to provide optimal care). In addition, during the exercise Karen's therapist learned that Karen was ignoring one of her major strengths as a health care provider—her sensitive and compassionate bedside manner. At first, Karen rejected this characteristic as having anything to do with competence. However, using Socratic questioning, Karen's therapist worked with her to see that a compassionate bedside manner might increase the likelihood that her patients would comply with their treatment regime, which would very much speak to her competence as a health care provider. At the end of the exercise, Karen decided that her compassionate bedside manner indeed contributes to her competence as a health care provider, and she re-rated herself at 70% on the competence-incompetence continuum.

3.7 Historical tests

Historical tests of unhelpful core beliefs allow patients to understand the pathway by which such beliefs developed, to examine evidence that supports and refutes the core beliefs at various periods of time in their life (e.g., elementary school years, middle school years, high school years, and so on), to reframe the evidence that they view as supportive the core beliefs, and to draw a more balanced conclusion that has direct implications for the core beliefs (J. S. Beck, 2011). This strategy was used with Gary, who distinctly remembered giving a presentation to his fourth grade class, when a classmate blurted out, "What's wrong with Gary? His face is all red." Gary identified the evidence that supported the core beliefs that he is weak and less than a man for several periods of his life, including elementary school, middle school, high school, college, and post-college. Gary identified several instances during each of these time periods that he viewed as supporting the unhelpful core beliefs, all of which involved becoming red and blotchy when he made presentations or asked young women out on dates. However, he also described many other accomplishments that had nothing to do with getting red and blotchy, such as being the captain of his high school soccer team and being accepted into a prestigious fraternity in college. He concluded that although he has had the propensity to turn red and blotchy throughout most of his life, he has received much recognition in his life that someone who is weak and less than a man would likely not have gotten.

3.8 Restructuring early memories

Therapists can use imagery and role-playing techniques in order to elicit affect associated with and restructure painful memories of events that shaped unhelpful core beliefs (J. S. Beck, 2011). Not only does completion of this exercise demonstrate to patients that their beliefs are understandable in light of their formative experiences, it also allows them to consider other explanations that might account for the unfortunate life events that contributed to them. Many approaches for implementing this strategy can be selected. In one application of this strategy, patients who present with distress about a current situation can think back to the first time they experienced similar distress and play the role of the person delivering the negative message in order to identify other explanations for that person's behavior. For example, Karen recalled that her father criticized her when she was in first grade because the neighbor boy got higher grades on his report card than she did, which gave her the message that she was inferior. Her therapist encouraged her to play the role of her father, and the therapist played the role of Karen when she was in first grade, responding to her "father" in a balanced manner. After completion of the role play, Karen realized that her father recognized her potential and wanted her to succeed because she was quite capable, rather than inferior.

Another application of this strategy involves a role-play between the patient at his or her current age and the patient at the age began to receive messages that contributed to the development of an unhelpful core belief. Such a role-play often begins with the therapist playing the role of the patient at that younger age, and the patient playing the role of the current him- or herself. The patient applies the cognitive restructuring skills that have been acquired in previous sessions to appraise the negative messages in a more balanced manner. Cori's therapist used this approach, inviting Cori to "show" her younger self that she has worth. Specifically, Cori's therapist made statements such as, "Well I am worthless. That's what Mommy and Daddy tell me. Cuz I always mess up things." In the context of the role-play, the adult Cori asked the younger Cori questions, such as, "Aren't kids allowed to mess up once in a while? How will you learn if you don't try? Does messing up something you are trying for the first time have to mean that you are worthless?" Later in the role-play, Cori assumed the role of her younger self, and her therapist played the role of her mother, telling her she was worthless. In her new role, the "young" Cori was encouraged to respond to her mother in a healthy, balanced manner, in which she stated, "Mommy, I'm just trying my best. Trying makes me worthwhile, not worthless." By "reliving" this experience, Cori was able to experience the intense affect associated with her mother's treatment of her and begin the reframe the hurtful message that she had internalized.

3.9 Defining the "new self"

Earlier in the chapter, I emphasized the importance of defining components of unhelpful core beliefs so that patients have an operational definition for their many components. In a similar manner, patients can define the precise operational components of their "new self" (D. Dobson & Dobson, 2009). In many instances, patients can translate their work on defining the unhelpful core belief to paint a picture of their "new self," developing goals they would like to achieve for each component. However, in other instances, patients are at a loss when they are asked to describe the person they would like to become and the associated healthy belief system. Thus, in these latter cases, patients can identify role models from biographies, movies, or the media and adopt the beliefs that these role models seem to expose.

For example, Marco's belief that he is not as good as other people often led him to "explode" at others when he perceived that he was being disrespected, which further reinforced his unhelpful core belief because he would chastise himself for not remaining "cooler" in challenging situations. He perceived the actor, George Clooney, to embody a healthy belief system that would, in turn, facilitate calm and centered responding in situations characterized by interpersonal conflict. Thus, he kept a mental image of George Clooney when he was faced with challenges, and when he successfully used this image to avert self-defeating behavior, his therapist helped him to use the experiences to reinforce his new, healthier belief that he is just as good as others.

3.10 Soliciting social support and consensus

Patients can also mobilize their social support system to help define and reinforce a new set of healthier core beliefs. Specifically, they can obtain feedback from others about the degree to which their old, unhealthy core beliefs are accurate, as well as about the proposed new, healthy set of core beliefs (D. Dobson & Dobson, 2009). Cori used this approach to address an intermediate belief, her attitude that being shy is perceived as a character defect (which, in turn, fueled her core belief that she is worthless). She constructed a questionnaire that she distributed to eight family members and friends, which was designed to solicit their feedback on the degree to which her shyness made a negative impact on her personality and behavior. She was shocked at the responses she received—although the family members and friends indeed acknowledged that they viewed her as shy, they, uniformly, did not regard her shyness as a character defect. Instead, they gave her the feedback that her quiet nature made her a good listener, and as a result, she was one of the first people they would go to when they needed support. Not only did this exercise refute the attitude that shyness was "bad," but it also refuted her core belief of worthlessness because she obtained evidence that other people valued her opinion.

3.11 Time projection

An approach for solidifying the adoption of a new, healthy belief system is *time projection*, in which patients create vivid images and descriptions of what life will be like at specific time periods in the future as a result of their new core beliefs. Creative ways to achieve time projection include having patients imaging writing a memoir at the end of their lives or a eulogy that captures how they would like to be remembered (D. Dobson & Dobson, 2009). These images and descriptions can then serve as a template to guide patients' appraisals of and behavior in new challenges that they face in their every day lives, such they are responding in a manner consistent with their new core beliefs, and more generally, the person they aspire to be. Toward the end of therapy, Gary used this approach to solidify his new core belief that he is a confident man with something to offer. He wrote a eulogy characterizing himself as a warm, funny, personable individual who had a wide social circle that valued and respected him. When he experienced the occasional twinge of anxiety about become red and blotchy while interaction with strangers, he recalled the spirit of the eulogy and was mindful that his warm interpersonal style was more salient than his redness and blotchiness, and that discontinuing the interaction would be contrary to the person by whom he wanted to be remembered.

4. Challenges and future directions

Many therapists find that working with core beliefs is quite rewarding, as it allows the therapist and patient to harness their creativity, it is intellectually stimulating, and it has the potential to facilitate lasting change in the patient. With those rewards, however, come potential challenges. Unhelpful core beliefs are often quite painful for patients to acknowledge, and sustained attention to core beliefs in session may be associated with an escalation of negative affect and agitation. Not only, then, is it important for the therapist to be comfortable in affective expression of this nature, but it is also imperative that the patient has coping skills in place to deal with the "side effects" of work with core beliefs (James & Barton, 2004). Because core beliefs are not modified fully after only one session, the patient may experience a temporary increase in symptoms in between sessions. Therapists should anticipate this and should work with patients to develop a specific cognitive behavioral coping plan to manage this affect.

In addition, there is no step-by-step procedure for working with core beliefs, in contrast to some cognitive therapy protocols that address situational automatic thoughts and behavioral coping skills. This is undoubtedly frustrating for the therapist-in-training who is learning how to administer cognitive therapy. In collaboration with their patients, therapists incorporate a variety of core belief modification strategies on the basis of the conceptualization of the patient's presenting problem, the factors that maintain or reinforce the core belief, and the patient's preferences. It is crucial for the therapist to keep in mind cognitive behavioral mechanisms of change, clearly map out the intended mechanism of the proposed strategy in light of this theory, and assess the degree to which the strategy achieved its anticipated outcome along the way. This approach reflects a true "scientist-practitioner" model of psychotherapy, such that relevant theory guides the choice of intervention, and the therapist collects "data" about the intervention to ensure that it is effective.

Although the efficacy and effectiveness of cognitive therapy, as a *treatment package*, have been evaluated in countless randomized controlled trials (Butler, Chapman, Forman, & Beck, 2006), rarely is research conducted to evaluate the effectiveness of particular cognitive therapy *strategies*. In fact, the research data have little to say about whether core belief work with patients even increases the efficacy of treatment above and beyond initial work with situational automatic thoughts, unhelpful behavioral patterns, and behavioral coping skills (D. Dobson & Dobson, 2009; see De Oliveira et al., in press, and Chapter 3 of this volume for an example of an exception). Thus, a much-needed direction for future research is to evaluate the efficacy of specific cognitive therapy strategies in reducing psychiatric symptoms, improving functioning, and improving quality of life. Such research would involve the time-series analysis of standardized assessments completed at the beginning and end of each therapy session, across the course of multiple sessions. Although it would be labor-intensive, such research would elucidate, more precisely, the short- and long-term effects of specific cognitive therapy strategies; clarify, more precisely, mechanisms of change; and speak to the ideal points in the course of cognitive therapy that specific strategies might be introduced. In other words, such research would move the field beyond the question of "Does cognitive therapy work" and toward the question of "How does cognitive therapy work?"

In conclusion, it is my speculation that work done early in the course of cognitive therapy, when therapists work with situational automatic thoughts, unhelpful behavioral patterns, and behavioral coping skills, is associated with substantial symptom reduction and increased motivation to make additional changes in therapy. For many patients, this is sufficient, and they are considered "treatment successes." However, it is also my speculation that the work done in the later sessions in therapy, when therapists work with core beliefs, is associated with enhanced consolidation of learning and relapse prevention, as well as shifts in cognitive and behavioral tendencies that underlie unhelpful personality styles. Although core belief work can be challenging for both the therapist and patient, it also can be some of the most gratifying work done in cognitive therapy due to its highly individualized and creative approach and its potential in creating lasting cognitive change in patients.

5. References

Amir, N., Beard, C., Burns, M., & Bomyea, J. (2009). Attention modification program in individuals with generalized anxiety disorder. *Journal of Abnormal Psychology, 118,* 28-33.

Amir, N., Beard, C., Taylor, C. T., Klumpp, H., Elias, J., Burns, M., et al. (2009). Attention training in individuals with generalized social phobia: A randomized controlled trial. *Journal of Consulting and Clinical Psychology, 77,* 961-973.

Beck, A. T. (1996). Beyond belief: A theory of modes, personality, and psychopathology. In P. Salkovskis (Ed.), *Frontiers of cognitive therapy* (pp. 1-25). New York, NY: Guilford.

Beck, A. T., & Beck, J. S. (1991). *The Personality Beliefs Questionnaire.* Unpublished assessment instrument. Beck Institute for Cognitive Therapy and Research, Bala Cynwyd, PA.

Beck, A. T., Butler, A. C., Brown, G. K., Dahlsgaard, K. K., Newman, C. F., & Beck, J. S. (2001). Dysfunctional beliefs discriminate personality disorders. *Behaviour Research and Therapy, 39,* 1213-1225.

Beck, A. T., Rush, A. J., Shaw, B. F., & Emery, G. (1979). *Cognitive therapy of depression.* New York, NY: Guilford Press.

Beck, J. S. (2011). *Cognitive behavior therapy: Basics and beyond (2nd ed.).* New York, NY: Guilford Press.

Bieling, P. J., Beck, A. T., & Brown, G. K. (2000). The Sociotropy-Autonomy Scale: Structure and implications. *Cognitive Therapy and Research, 24,* 763-780.

Burns, D. D. (1980). *Feeling good: The new mood therapy.* New York, NY: Signet.

Butler, A. C., Chapman, J. E., Forman, E. M., & Beck, A. T. (2006). The empirical status of cognitive-behavioral therapy: a review of meta-analyses. *Clinical Psychology Review, 26,* 17-31.

Clark, D. A., & Beck, A. T. (1999). *Scientific foundations of cognitive theory and therapy of depression*. New York, NY: Wiley.

De Oliveira, I. R., Powell, V. B., Wenzel, A., Caldas, M., Seixas, C., Almeida, C., et al. (in press). Efficacy of the Trial-Based Thought Record: A new cognitive therapy strategy designed to change core beliefs in social phobia. *Journal of Clinical Pharmacy and Therapeutics*.

Dobson, D., & Dobson, K. S. (2009). *Evidence-based practice of cognitive-behavioral therapy*. New York, NY: Guilford Press.

Dobson, K. S. (2012). *Cognitive therapy*. Washington, DC: APA Books.

James, I. A., & Barton, S. (2004). Changing core beliefs with the continuum technique. *Behavioural and Cognitive Psychotherapy, 32*, 431-442.

Weissman, A. N., & Beck, A. T. (1980). *The Dysfunctional Attitudes Scale*. Unpublished Manuscript, University of Pennsylvania, Philadelphia, PA.

Wenzel, A., Brown, G. K., & Karlin, B. E. (2011). *Cognitive behavioral therapy for depressed Veterans and Military servicemembers: Therapist manual*. Washington, DC: U.S. Department of Veterans Affairs.

Part 2

Cognitive-Behavioral Therapy

4

Cognitive-Behavioral Therapy for Depression*

Neander Abreu[1], Vania Bitencourt Powell[2] and Donna Sudak[3]
[1]*Institute of Psychology, Federal University of Bahia, Salvador,*
[2]*Post-Graduation Program, Department of Neuroscience and Mental Health,*
Professor Edgard Santos University Hospital, Federal University of Bahia, Salvador,
[3]*Department of Psychiatry, Drexel University, Philadelphia,*
[1,2]*Brazil*
[3]*USA*

1. Introduction

Depression has a substantial impact on the lives of patients and their families, significantly affecting their social and occupational lives as well as causing other functional impairments (Murray & Lopez, 1996).

The objective of this chapter is to present the use of cognitive-behavioral therapy (CBT) in patients with depression by describing the techniques used and the efficacy of this therapeutic strategy. To achieve this aim, a search was accomplished to identify the principal relevant clinical trials by conducting a non-systematic literature review using the Medline, SciELO and PsychInfo databases, supplemented with textbooks on the subject. A description of the CBT model is followed by a discussion on efficacy studies.

2. Epidemiological aspects

Major depressive episode (MDE) is one of the most prevalent psychiatric disorders. A study carried out in the United States using the DSM-IV (American Psychiatric Association, 1996) criteria reported lifetime prevalence of 16.2%, and 12-month prevalence of 6.6% (Kessler et al., 2003).

For many patients, the disorder is chronic and recurrent. Follow-up studies have shown that up to 30% of patients remain depressed after one year, 18% after two years and 12% after five years. Many treated patients retain residual and subsyndromal symptoms that are associated with unfavorable outcomes such as higher risk of recurrence and suicide, poorer psychosocial functioning and elevated mortality resulting from clinical diseases. Of the patients who recover from a depressive episode, more than 50% relapse (Kennedy et al., 2004). The return of depressive symptoms during maintenance therapy with antidepressants occurs at rates that vary from 9 to 57% (Byrne & Rothschild, 1998).

The greatest concern in the follow-up of these patients is suicide, which is significantly associated with major depression. Based on the results of a meta-analysis, the estimated risk

---

*This chapter is an update of Powell et al.'s (2008) article.

of suicide was 2.2% in less severe outpatients and 8.6% in those with more severe depression and a history of hospitalization (Bostwick & Pankratz, 2000). Because of its high prevalence and resulting disability (major depression is classified as the second greatest cause of disability, adjusted for years of life, in developed countries) (Murray & Lopez, 1996). The concern in preventing recurrences of MDE is relevant and has been the target of research both with pharmacological treatment and psychotherapy (Antonuccio et al., 1995; Fava et al., 1996; Fava et al., 1998a; Fava et al., 1998b; Hollon et al., 2005).

3. The cognitive model and depression

In the 1960s, Albert Ellis and Aaron Beck reached the important conclusion that depression was the result of extremely deeply established thought habits, and described the fundamental concepts of cognitive-behavioral therapy. Beck (1963; 1967) observed that negative moods and behavior were usually the result of distorted thoughts and beliefs and not of unconscious forces, as the Freudian theory suggested. In other words, depression may be understood as being the result of the patient's own cognitions and dysfunctional cognitive strategies. Patients with depression believe and act as if things were worse than they really are. This new treatment approach emphasizing thought was referred to by Beck as cognitive therapy (Beck, 1963). To this date, more than 300 controlled clinical trials have confirmed the efficacy of this therapy, which makes it the psychotherapeutic option with the greatest empirical support (Beck, 2005; Butler et al., 2006).

As developed by Aaron T. Beck, cognitive behavioral therapy (CBT) for depression is currently the best-researched therapeutic strategy for any psychological disorder (Beck, 2005). Many studies and meta-analyses have confirmed its efficacy for the treatment of mild, moderate or severe depression. Furthermore, CBT is at least as effective as pharmacological therapy or any other form of psychological intervention [e.g. interpersonal therapy (IPT) or supportive treatment] (Dobson, 1989). An additional benefit of CBT has been recorded in many treatment studies; it results in a more durable response compared to drug therapy and may be protective against recurrence (Hollon et al., 2005; Hollon et al., 1991).

4. Cognitive triad

Beck's cognitive theory of depression assumes two basic elements: the cognitive triad and cognitive distortions (Beck, 1963). The cognitive triad consists of a negative vision of oneself in which the person tends to see him/herself as inadequate or inept (e.g. "*I am a boring person*", "*I am uninteresting*", "*I am too sad for anyone to like me*"), a negative view of the world, including relationships, work and activities (e.g. "*No one appreciates my job*") and a negative view of the future, which appears to be cognitively linked to the degree of hopelessness. The most typical thoughts and verbal expressions with respect to a negative view of the future include: "*Things are never going to get any better*", "*I will never be worth anything*" or "*I'll never be happy*". Such thoughts, when coupled with hopelessness and suicidal ideation may make death seem like a relief from psychological pain or suffering or an escape from a situation perceived to be unbearable (Beck, 1976).

Beck et al. (1979) observed that the depressed patients describe their experience negatively and expect unfavorable outcomes to occur. This manner of interpreting events and expectations makes inactivity and inertia seem logical, which in turn, serves to reinforce the depressed person's feelings of inadequacy, low self-esteem and hopelessness.

5. Cognitive distortions

Cognitive distortions, defined as systematic errors in the perception and processing of information, occupy a central role in depression. Individuals with depression tend to be absolute and inflexible in structuring their experiences, leading to errors of interpretation with regard to personal performance and judgment of external situations (J. S. Beck 1995; Scher et al., 2006).

The most common cognitive distortions in depressed patients were classified by Beck et al. (1979) into a typological system that includes, among others, arbitrary inference (formulating a conclusion in the absence of sufficient evidence), selective abstraction (tendency of the person to select proof of his/her poor performance), overgeneralization (tendency to consider that one negative event or performance will occur other times), and personalization (personal attribution, often negative). A larger series of distortions has been described by Beck and others (Beck et al., 1979; Scher et al., 2006). Recently, de-Oliveira (chapter 1) developed the Cognitive Distortions Questionnaire (CD-Quest), a questionnaire to help therapist and patient to assess and follow changes in cognitive distortions frequency and intensity during therapy.

Cognitive distortions logically follow the patient's internal rules and assumptions, which are stable patterns of thinking developed throughout the lifetime of every individual. These rules and beliefs are sensitive to activation by primary sources such as stress or losses and often lead to ineffective interpersonal strategies (Scher et al., 2006).

6. Use of cognitive therapy in depression

Cognitive therapy for depression is a treatment process that helps patients alter beliefs and behaviors that produce certain mood states. The therapeutic strategies of cognitive-behavioral management of depression occur in three phases: 1) education, forming the therapeutic relationship and making behavioral changes to confront problems with poor self-care and vegetative symptoms; 2) focus on automatic thoughts; and 3) focus on dysfunctional core beliefs.

One of the advantages of cognitive therapy is the way in which patients actively participate in their own treatment, helping them to: a) identify distorted perceptions; b) recognize negative thoughts and seek alternative thoughts that more closely reflect reality; c) find evidence supporting negative and alternative thoughts; and d) generate more believable and accurate thoughts associated with certain situations in a process called cognitive restructuring; d) behave in more functional ways; and e) manage life problems more effectively (Beck, 1979).

7. Behavioral activation

One of the theories that guides the procedures involved in the treatment of depression is Lewinsohn's (1974, 1975) theory that social learning and the level of positive reinforcement are factors that contribute towards the onset and maintenance of depressive states. This theory states that patients become depressed because they are experiencing a decrease in the general reinforcement they receive from the outside world – as a result of a decreased positive reinforcement and/or an excess of aversive experiences. Depression is conceived in this model as a vicious circle in which the patient gradually withdraws from positive activities and experiences the exponential loss of positive reinforcement. Therefore, the therapist must work incisively to increase the involvement of depressed patients in activities that should result in positive reinforcement and social interaction.

The behavioral strategies used in CBT originate from Lewinsohn's (1974, 1975) model of psychopathology and are used flexibly. These strategies are planned in accordance with each individual patient and are used in such a way as to engage the patient, relieve symptoms and obtain information that is relevant to therapy.

The initial strategy, consisting of the scheduling and monitoring of activities, is a powerful tool to be used by patients with depression. In fact, some patients with depression may respond to behavioral activation alone (Dimidjian et al., 2006). The scheduling of activities may be used flexibly by clinicians and patients to monitor activities (to correct distortions in the way patients think they are spending their time and to evaluate activities associated with control and pleasure), to schedule enjoyable activities and productive activities (particularly for depressed patients who do not allow themselves to participate in these activities) and to identify activities related to very positive or very negative feelings. This technique provides the patient and the therapist with data on how the patient is functioning. Scheduling of activities may be used to plan behavioral tasks and to record results. Acting according to a plan rather than waiting for a "feeling" is much more effective for depressed patients. Moreover, this procedure gives patients control over their time, recognizes their efforts with respect to performing activities and records true accomplishments. This technique is a powerful tool to be used with patients under pharmacological treatment, since it will give them the opportunity to record side effects, activities and changes in symptoms. This relatively simple intervention can illustrate the relationship between depressive symptoms and lack of intentional, positive behaviors, thereby opening a pathway towards solving problems (Beck et al., 1979).

In CBT, skill deficits are also conceptualized as factors that may contribute to the risk for depression. For example, if the individual is unable to be assertive in interpersonal relationships, he/she misses out on an important opportunity for positive reinforcement. One significant contribution of Beck and other investigators to this model is the idea that, besides the reduction in positive reinforcement, depressed patients also increase the magnitude of their symptoms through the cognitive evaluations and conclusions that they reach from the lack of positive reinforcement. For example, depressed patients carry out fewer and fewer activities and conclude that it is hopeless to try and do anything. When therapists help patients modify this behavior, this brings direct evidence that their cognitive evaluations are incorrect. Patients then have a powerful example of how errors in their way of thinking have led to dysfunctional emotions and behavioral responses, and the treatment advances by cognitive and behavioral means to solving problems (Sudak, 2006).

8. Cognitive restructuring

The initial sessions are also directed towards defining the patients' problems by elaborating the conceptualization or formulation of the case. In these sessions, therapists will help patients identify: 1) the particular dysfunctional beliefs they have associated with depression; 2) their most common cognitive distortions and classification of automatic thoughts; 3) the physiological, emotional and behavioral reactions arising from these thoughts; 4) behaviors that were developed to confront dysfunctional beliefs; and 5) how previous experiences have contributed towards maintaining the patients' beliefs (J. S. Beck, 1995).

8.1 Evoking thoughts and assumptions

Depression generates immobility and pessimism; therefore, patients find it difficult to begin any task and fail to identify any advantage in performing any activity. An initial step in treating patients, following behavioral activation is to help the patient to identify such thoughts.

Of note, the goal of cognitive therapy in MDE is to facilitate the remission of depression and to teach patients to be their own therapists. Cognitive techniques should help achieve the objectives of therapy and should be understood by the patient as tools that they can use in the future. Patients should be stimulated to confront the problems related to mood complaints and therapists should not help them with each problem, since this may prevent strengthening their own abilities (Beck et al., 1979). An extensive series of cognitive techniques and the discussion of their applications may be found in Leahy's excellent textbook (Leahy, 2003). Some of the techniques that have proven more effective in the treatment of MDE are presented below.

8.2 Explanation on how thoughts are related to feelings

A direct question by the therapist such as *"what were you thinking about at that moment?"* or *"what went through your mind right now?"* when the patient exhibits a shift in emotion or relays an emotionally-laden situation, may be supplemented by a table with two parallel columns describing: 1) I think that ...; and 2) Hence, I feel... When the therapist uses this type of resource, difficulties may arise for the patient to correctly identify thoughts and feelings, and the therapist's help may be necessary (Leahy, 2003).

8.3 Recording dysfunctional thoughts

This technique increases objectivity and encourages the individual to remember events, thoughts and feelings that occurred between sessions. Generally, the individual needs training to use this daily thought diary, initially being able to identify automatic thoughts by first identifying emotional states. The tool comprises a register in which the patient writes down sequentially an event and the subsequent thought that occurs at a time of problematic emotions or behaviors. There is an additional column to give a note related to what extent the patient believes that thought is true. This column will progressively help the individual identify which dysfunctional automatic thoughts are most likely to be a productive focus of attention. Next, the emotion is recorded and the degree of emotion is evaluated on a 0-10 or

0-100 scale. To help the patient, comparison may be made with the most intense emotion (sadness, for example) in order to reach a more realistic evaluation (Beck et al., 1979). Thought records also include an evidence-gathering column, and a column to generate an alternative thought about the situation. Finally, the patient is asked to rate the believability of the new thought as well as to rate the intensity of the emotion (Padesky & Greenberger, 1995).

8.4 Trial-Based Thought Record (TBTR)

De Oliveira (2008) has developed the TBTR, a 7-column thought record designed to address core beliefs by means of sentence-reversion and the analogy to a judicial process. This method might be useful in restructuring negative beliefs in depressed patients. Despite the lack of clinical trials comparing this method with other psychological approaches used to treat depression, case reports indicate its potential in this regard. The inspiration for its development came from the surreal novel by Franz Kafka, *The Trial* (Kafka, 1998; first published in 1925). The rational basis to propose the TBTR is that it could be useful to make patients aware of their core beliefs about themselves (self-accusations) and engage them in a constructive trial to develop more positive and functional core beliefs (De-Oliveira, 2011). TBTR incorporates a structured format and sequentially presents several techniques already used in conventional cognitive therapy: downward arrow technique, examining the evidence, defense attorney technique, thought reversal, upward arrow technique, developing a more positive schema, and positive self-statement logs, and the empty chair approach (see chapter 3 in this book).

8.5 Downward arrow

As patients become more capable of identifying and restructuring automatic thoughts, it is important to investigate the underlying beliefs that lead to such thoughts, and make the person vulnerable to negative events. Changing such beliefs increases the durability of recovery from depression (DeRubeis et al., 1990; Hollon et al., 1990).

A form of Socratic questioning called downward arrow can be used to help identify such beliefs about the self and others (Burns, 1980; De-Oliveira, 2011). The Socratic method is also used to help the patient develop autonomous reasoning to question the evidence and create alternative thoughts and evaluations. Confronting the evidence of thoughts may help patients reduce the power of the thought, decreasing their feelings of fear, sadness or discouragement. The downward arrow is a very useful technique that helps to oppose beliefs that maintain the state of depression.

9. The duration of treatment and remission of symptoms

Although patients with axis 2 co-morbidity or significant anxiety symptoms associated with depression may require longer treatment with cognitive therapy, this therapy normally is short-term (Blenkiron, 1999). Structured sessions also help patients develop a sense of personal control and enhance the efficiency of treatment. Patients with personality disorders may require more time in therapy, even more than 12 months (Byrne & Rothschild, 1998). Often, these patients tend to drop out from treatment more easily and the therapist should be attuned to the therapeutic alliance. Some research has indicated the patients with Axis 2 disorders who cannot receive longer courses of CBT might benefit more from managing symptoms with medication (Fournier et al., 2008), or behavioral activation (Coffman et al., 2007).

In addition, the therapist should also be attentive that patients may drop out or interrupt their treatment following the remission of the first symptoms that had previously maintained them less active and less confident. As these symptoms improve, there may be a tendency to drop out treatment prematurely.

10. Prevention of relapses

The final sessions are aimed at evaluating the advances made in therapy and at preventing recurrences. The patient's improvement may be used as a resource for confronting new situations that include losses and adaptations to current problems. From the beginning, it should be emphasized that the duration of therapy is limited; the procedures involved in therapy should be demystified by relating them to the identification of thoughts, their questioning and restructuring; the patients' confidence should be increased based on their gains; and, gradually patients increase their role in the process of change. All these procedures facilitate progress towards the termination of therapy and generate confidence in patients to proceed with their lives. The therapist must teach patients to deal with the possibility of a recurrence of depressive symptoms, since depression is a highly recurrent disorder (Deckrsbach et al., 2000).Therefore, another important strength of cognitive therapy is its durability in recurrent unipolar depression, as compared to pharmacological treatments (Fava et al., 1998).

Fava et al. (1996) suggested that cognitive therapy for the residual symptoms of a depressive episode treated with medication leads to substantially fewer recurrences. In a preliminary study involving 40 patients, those with recurrent major depression who had been successively treated with antidepressants were randomly allocated into two groups, one treated with cognitive therapy for the residual symptoms and the other with conventional clinical management. After 20 weeks of treatment, the administration of antidepressants was reduced and then ceased in both groups. Patients were followed up for two years during which no medication was used except for cases of recurrence. The group in which cognitive therapy was given was found to have significantly fewer residual symptoms compared to the group that received conventional clinical management. Cognitive therapy also resulted in lower recurrence rates (25%) compared to clinical management (80%).

Data referring to the patients of the above-mentioned study were published after 4 and 6 years of follow-up (Fava et al., 1998a; Fava et al., 1998b). Treatment with cognitive therapy resulted in a significant reduction in recurrence rates at 4 years (35% versus 70%) (Fava et al., 1998a). After 6 years of follow-up (Fava et al., 1998b), 10 of the patients in the cognitive therapy group (50%) and 15 of the patients in conventional treatment (75%) had suffered relapses; however, this difference was not statistically significant. When multiple recurrences were considered, the patients submitted to cognitive therapy had significantly fewer episodes and responded to the same antidepressant used in the basal episode of the study. The authors concluded that cognitive therapy seems to offer a protective effect for up to four years of follow-up, and this effect becomes weaker afterwards. Nevertheless, cognitive therapy for the residual symptoms led to a long-term reduction in the number of episodes of major depression (Fava et al., 1998a). According to Fava et al. (1998b), these results challenge the established belief that prolonged pharmacological treatment is the only way of preventing relapses in patients with recurrent depression.

However, in what way would CBT prevent recurrences in patients with MDE? One proposal denominated "metacognitive awareness" may explain this phenomenon. Instead of considering the modification of dysfunctional beliefs as a tool for preventing recurrences, the metacognitive awareness approach suggests that the negative thoughts and feelings in MDE are experienced as mental events and not as an expression of reality. As patients evolve in their depressive state, they cease to automatically accept the negative thoughts. This hypothesis, still under investigation, seems useful as an explanation for the success achieved with cognitive therapy in the prevention of recurrences.

Another study (Murphy et al., 1984) followed patients with MDE for two years. Patients who had had a mean of three episodes of moderate to severe MDE were divided into three treatment groups: 1) antidepressants (AD); 2) CBT with monthly maintenance; and 3) AD in the acute phase plus CBT with monthly maintenance. Patients were distributed as follows: AD: 31%; monthly CBT: 36%; AD + monthly CBT: 24%. At the end of 24 months, there was no statistically significant difference in recurrence rates. This study showed that cognitive therapy was at least as effective as AD in maintaining remission and preventing relapses. Maintenance pharmacotherapy may be necessary for some patients while cognitive therapy is a viable alternative for others.

11. Cognitive therapy and pharmacotherapy

The first study on CBT for depression was published in 1977 (Rush et al., 1977). The authors compared CBT to imipramine and reported significantly better results with CBT. This study was not, however, placebo controlled. Another significant limitation was that the research team was not blinded with respect to the form of treatment, so further investigation was necessary to confirm efficacy. By 1989, a sufficient number of studies had been performed to allow a review and meta-analysis to be carried out (Dobson, 1989). Twenty-eight studies were included in that sample, which found better results for CBT compared to medication and other psychological treatments. In subsequent years, various studies confirmed the significant efficacy of CBT in the treatment of major depression and its increased durability compared to pharmacological therapy. The sole exception to this was the NIMH's Treatment of Depression Collaborative Research Project (TDCRP), a large, multi-centered trial of CBT versus IPT versus medication (imipramine) versus placebo. CBT performed as well as IPT/imipramine in cases of mild to moderate depression, but in cases of more severe depression, IPT and imipramine gave better results (Elkin et al., 1989). Further analysis carried out by DeRubeis et al. (1999) on the data from this study indicated that there were significant differences in the efficacy of CBT across sites. In Philadelphia, where therapist fidelity to the model was more robust, CBT performed as well as IPT or medication. DeRubeis and Feeley subsequently studied therapist fidelity to the model and found that therapist fidelity early in treatment is predictive of patient response in depression.

Following TDCRP (Elkin et al., 1989), a significant number of studies went on to expand the empirical basis for the use of CBT in acute and chronic depression, both alone and in combination with medication (Jarrett et al., 1999; Hollon et al., 1992). Many studies evaluating efficacy were conducted in order to establish CBT as being at least as effective as or superior to a pharmacological intervention. Greenberg and Fisher (1997, 1989) described a number of well-conducted clinical trials comparing active and directive psychotherapies (such as cognitive and interpersonal therapies) with antidepressants and suggested that outpatients submitted to psychotherapy evolved just as well or at times better than those receiving medication. They also concluded that, although medication improved sleep-related symptoms, psychotherapy was more effective in helping patients with depression and apathy. Moreover, unlike psychotherapy, medication was unable to help depressed outpatients to adjust socially, and to recover their interpersonal relationships and their professional performance (De-Oliveira, 1998).

Systematic reviews and meta-analyses have noted that CBT has efficacy similar to that of antidepressant treatment (Dobson, 1989; Hollon et al., 1991; Conte et al., 1986; Robinson et al., 1990; Wexler & Cicchetti, 1992). Treatment with psychotherapy also conveyed an advantage with respect to dropout rates and recurrences (de Jonghe, 2001). Another large clinical trial (Keller et al., 2000) was conducted with 681 patients with chronic and recurrent major nonpsychotic depression, and compared nefazodone, cognitive behavioral-analysis system of psychotherapy (a recently developed form of cognitive therapy), and the combination thereof. A total of 16-20 sessions were conducted over 12 weeks. Taking into consideration only patients who completed the study, remission or a satisfactory response was achieved in 85% of cases in the group that received the combined treatment and in 55% of cases in the group treated with nefazodone or therapy alone.

Most combined treatment studies accomplished to date are heterogeneous regarding the medications evaluated and did not employ adequate pharmacotherapy as implemented in clinical practice; hence, it is difficult to draw adequate conclusions with respect to the added benefits of combined treatment versus the use of either modality alone. Nevertheless, several reviews and one interesting meta-analysis indicate that in cases of more severe depression there may be a significant added benefit with the combined use of medication and cognitive behavioral treatments (Hollon et al., 1991; Friedman et al., 2006). Several studies have been conducted to counter the objections raised about data acquired in earlier studies of CBT for depression. Most impressively, DeRubeis et al. (2005) published a definitive study comparing CBT to medication, which included a placebo control group and an augmentation protocol for non-responders to the initial study medication. This study included patients who were moderately to severely depressed, and who had co-morbid anxiety and personality disorders. CBT and medication performed equally well for the acute treatment of moderate to severe depression.

As previously discussed, the most impressive finding in studies of CBT for depression is the durability of its effect. Patients who are CBT responders have a significantly more durable response than patients whose depression is treated with medication. Many recent reviews describe substantial decrement in response to antidepressant medication even if the patient continues taking the medication properly, an event that occurs only 26% of the time (Bockting et al., 2008).

Recurrence of major depression is common. Several studies have attempted to forestall this recurrence by employing novel strategies in CBT. Jarrett et al. (1999) have shown that booster sessions of CBT have a substantial effect on the recurrence of depression in chronic patients who are CBT responders. Several studies have evaluated the sequential treatment with medication and CBT using a brief CBT protocol applied either individually or in groups following treatment with medication, including Fava's studies previously described (Fava et al., 1998a; Fava et al., 1998b; Fava et al., 1998; Bockting et al., 2008 and Paykel et al. (1999) achieved similarly impressive results using individual and group treatment strategies with a very short-term treatment protocol. Mindfulness-based cognitive therapy has also been successfully used in chronic depression to forestall recurrence after successful remission has been achieved (Teasdale et al., 2000).

In conclusion, CBT in the treatment of depression is one of the therapeutic alternatives with the highest empirical evidence of efficacy, whether applied alone or in combination with pharmacotherapy.

12. References

American Psychiatric Association (1994). *Diagnostic and statistical manual of mental disorders* (DSM-IV). 4th edition. Washington (DC): American Association.

American Psychiatric Association() (2000). *Diagnostic and statistical manual of disorders* (DSM-IV-TR). 4th Edition Text Revision. Washington (DC): American Psychiatric Association.

Antonuccio DO, Danton WG, DeNelsky GY () (1995) . Psychotherapy versus Medication for depression: challenging the conventional wisdom with data. *Prof Psychol Res Pract,,* 26(6):574-85.

Beck AT (1976). *Cognitive therapy and the emotional disorders.* Boston: International University Press.

Beck AT (1967). *Depression: causes and treatment.* Philadelphia: University of Pennsylvania Press.

Beck AT (2005). The current state of cognitive therapy: a 40-year retrospective. *Arch Gen Psychiatry, ,* 62(9):953-9.

Beck AT (1963). *Thinking and depression.* Arch Gen Psychiatry,, 9:324-33.

Beck AT, Rush AJ, Shaw BF, Emery G (1979). *Cognitive Therapy of Depression.* New York: Guilford Press.

Beck JS (1995) (1995). *Cognitive therapy: basics and beyond.* New York: Guilford Press.

Blackburn IM, Eunson KM, Bishop S (1986). A 2-year naturalistic follow-up of patients treated with cognitive therapy, pharmacotherapy and a combination of both. *J Affect Disord.,* 10(1):67-75.

Blenkiron P (1999). Who is suitable for cognitive therapy behavioural therapy? *J R Soc Med.,* 92(5):222-9.

Bockting C, ten Doesschate MC, Spijker J, Spinhoven P, Koeter MW, Schene AH (2008): DELTA Study Group. Continuation and maintenance use of antidepressants in recurrent depression. *Psychother Psychosom.,* 77(1):17-26

Bostwick JM, Pankratz VS (2000). Affective disorders and suicide risk: a reexamination. *Am J Psychiatry,* 157(12):1925-32.

Butler AC, Chapman JE, Forman EM, Beck AT (2006). The empirical status of cognitive-behavioral therapy: a review of meta-analyses. *Clin Psychol Rev.,* 26(1):17-31.

Burns DD (1980). *Feeling good: the new mood therapy.* New York: Signet.1980.

Byrne SE, Rothschild AJ (1998). Loss of antidepressant efficacy during Maintenance therapy: possible mechanisms and treatments. *J Clin Psychiatry.* 59(6):279-88.

Coffman, S.J., Martell, C.R., Dimidjian, S., et al (2007). Extreme nonresponse in therapy: Can behavioral activation succeed where cognitive therapy fails. *Journal of Consulting and Clinical Psychology,* 75(4): 531-541.

Conte HR, Plutchik R, Wild KV, Karasu TB (1986). Combined psychotherapy and pharmacotherapy for depression. A systematic analysis of the evidence. *Arch Gen Psychiatry.* 1986;43(5):471-9.

Deckrsbach T, Gershuny BS, Otto MW (2000). Cognitive-behavioral therapy for depression. *Psychiatr Clin North Am.,* 23(4):795-809.

de Jonghe F, Kool S, van Aalst G, Dekker J, Peen J (2001). Combining psychotherapy and antidepressants in the treatment of depression. *J Affect Dis.* 2001;64(2-3):217-29.

De-Oliveira IR (2011). Kafka´s trial dilemma: proposal of a practical solution to Joseph K.´s unknown accusation. *Medical Hypotheses,* 77, 5-6.

De-Oliveira IR (2008). Trial-Based Thought Record (TBTR): preliminary data on a strategy to deal with core beliefs by combining sentence reversion and the use of analogy with a judicial process. *Rev Bras Psiquiatr.,* 30(1):12-8.

De-Oliveira IR (2007). Sentence-reversion-based thought record (SRBTR): a new strategy to deal with "yes, but..." dysfunctional thoughts in cognitive therapy. *Eur Rev Appl Psychol.,* 57:17-22.

De-Oliveira IR (2011) Kafka's trial dilemma: proposal of a practical solution to Joseph K.'s unknown accusation. Medical Hypotheses, 77, 5–6.

DeRubeis RJ, Feeley M (1990). Determinants of change in cognitive therapy for depression. *Cog Ther Res.,* 14:464-82.

DeRubeis RJ, Gelfand LA, Tang TZ, Simons AD (1999). Medications versus cognitive-behavioral therapy for severely depressed outpatients: mega- analysis of four randomized comparisons. *Am J Psychiatry.,* 156(7): 1007-13.

DeRubeis RJ, Hollon SD, Amsterdam JD, Shelton RC, Young PR, Saloman RM, O'Reardon JP, Lovett ML, Gladis MM, Brown LL, Gallop R (2005). Cognitive therapy vs medications in the treatment of moderate to severe depression. *Arch Gen Psychiatry,,* 62(4):409-16.

Dimidjian S., Hollon, S.D., Dobson, S., et al (2006). Randomized trial of behavioral activation, cognitive therapy, and antidepressant medication in the acute treatment of adults with major depression. *Journal of Consulting and Clinical Psychology.,* 74(4): 658-670.

Dobson KS (1989). A meta-analysis of the efficacy of cognitive therapy for depression. *J Consult Clin Psychol.* , 57(3):414-9.

Elkin I, Shea MT, Watkins JT, Imber SD, Sotsky SM, Collins JF, Glass DR, Pilokins PA, Leber WR, Docerty JP (1989). National Institute of Mental Health treatment of depression collaborative research program. General effectiveness of treatments. *Arch Gen Psychiatry,* 46(11):971-82.

Fava GA, Grandi S, Zielezny M, Rafanelli C, Canestrari R (1996). Four-year outcome for cognitive behavioral treatment of residual symptoms in major depression. *Am J Psychiatry,* 153(7):945-7.

Fava GA, Rafanelli C, Grandi S, Canestrari R, Morphy MA (1998a). Six-year outcome for cognitive behavioral treatment of residual symptoms in major depression. *Am J Psychiatry*, 155(10):1443-5.

Fava GA, Rafanelli C, Grandi S, Conti S, Belluardo P (1998b). Prevention of recurrent depression with cognitive behavioral therapy: preliminary findings. *Arch Gen Psychiatry*, 55(9):816-20.

Fournier, J.C., DeRubeis, R.J., Shelton, R.C., et al (2008). Antidepressant medications vs. cognitive therapy in people with or without personality disorder. *British Journal of Psychiatry*, 192: 124-129

Freeman A, DeWolf R (1992) (1992). The 10 *dumbest mistakes smart people make and how to avoid them*. New York: Harper Perennial.

Friedman ES, Wright JH, Jarrett RB, Thase ME (2006). Combining cognitive therapy and medication for mood disorders. *Psychiatr Ann.*, 36: 320-8.

Greenberg, RP, Fisher S (1989). Examining antidepressant effectiveness: findings, ambiguities, and some vexing puzzles. In: Fisher S, Greenberg RP, editors. *The limits of biological treatments for psychological distress*. Hillsdale (NJ): Erlbaum.

Greenberg RP, Fisher S (1997). Mood mending medicines: probing drug, psychotherapy and placebo solutions. In: Fisher S, Greenberg RP, editors. *From placebo to panacea: putting psychiatric drugs to the test*. New York: John Wiley & Sons.

Hollon, S.D., Evans, M.D., DeRubeis, R.J (1990). Cognitive Mediation of Relapse Prevention Following Treatment for Depression: Implications of Differential Risk In Psychological Aspects of Depression. In Ingram RE, Editor: *Contemporary psychological approaches to depression*. New York: Plenum,, pp. 117-136.

Hollon SD, DeRubeis RJ, Evans MD, Wiemer MY, Garvey MS, Grove WM, Tuason VB (1992). Cognitive therapy and pharmacoptherapy for depression. Singly and in combination. *Arch Gen Psychiatry*, 49 (10):774-81.

Hollon SD, Jarrett RB, Nierenberg AA, Thase ME, Trivedi M, Rush AJ (2005). Psychotherapy and medication in the treatment of adult and geriatric depression: which monotherapy or combined treatment? *J Clin Psychiatry*. 2005;66(4):455-68.

Hollon SD, Shelton RC, Loosen PT (1991). Cognitive therapy and pharmacotherapy for depression. *J Consult Clin Psychol.*, 59(1): 88-99.

Jarrett RB, Schaffer M, McIntire D, Witt-Browder A, Kraft D, Risser RC (1999). Treatment of atypical depression with cognitive therapy or phenelzine. *Arch Gen Psychiatry*, 56:431-7.

Kafka F (1998). *The trial*. New York: Schocken.

Keller MB, McCullough JP, Klein DN, Arnow B, Dunner DL, Gelenberg AJ, Markowitz JC, Nemeroff CB, Russell JM, Thase ME, Trivedi MH, Zajecka J (2000). A comparison of nefazodone, the cognitive behavioral-analysis system of psychotherapy, and their combination for the treatment of chronic depression. *N Eng J Med.*, 342:1462-70.

Kennedy SH, Lam RW, Nutt DJ, Thase ME (2004). Psychotherapies, alone and in combination. In: Kennedy SH, Lam RW, Nutt DJ, Thase ME, editors. *Treating depression effectively: applying clinical guidelines*. London: Martin Dunitz.

Kessler RC, Berglund P, Demler O, Jin R, Koretz D, Merikangas KR, Rush AJ, Walters EE, Wang PS (2003). National Comorbidity Survey Replication. The epidemiology of major depressive disorder: results from the National. Comorbidity Survey Replication (NCS-R). *JAMA*, 289(23): 3095-105.

Klein D (1995). Diagnosis and classification of dysthymic disorder. In: Kocsis JH, Klein DN, editors. *Diagnosis and treatment of chronic depression*. New York: Guilford.

Leahy RL (2003). *Cognitive therapy techniques: a practitioner's guide*. New York: Guilford Press.

Lewinsohn PM (1974). A behavioral approach to depression. In: Friedman RM, Katz MM, editors. *The psychology of depression*. Contemporary theory and research. Washington, DC: Winston-Wiley.

Lewinsohn PM (1975). The behavioral study and treatment of depression. In: Hersen M, Eisler RM, Miller PM, editors. *Progress in behavior modification*. Vol. 1. New York: Academic Press.

Murphy GE, Simons AD, Wetzel RD, Lustman PJ (1984). Cognitive therapy and pharmacotherapy. Singly and together in the treatment of depression. *Arch Gen Psychiatry*, ;41(1):33-41.

Murray CJ, Lopez AD, editors (1996). *The global burden of disease series*. Boston, MA: Harvard School of Public Health.

Padesky CA, Greenberger D (1995). *Clinician's guide to mind over mood*. New York: Guilford Press.

Paykel ES, Scott J, Teasdale JD, Johnson AL, Garland A, Moore R, Jenaway A, Cornwall PL, Hayhurst H, Abbott R, Pope M (1999). Prevention of relapse in residual depression by cognitive therapy. *Arch Gen Psychiatry*, 56(9):829-35.

Powell VB, Abreu N, de Oliveira IR, Sudak D (2008). Cognitive-behavioral therapy for depression. *Rev Bras Psiquiatr.*, 30(Suppl II):S73-80

Robinson LA, Berman JS, Neimeyer RA (1990). Psychotherapy for the treatment of depression: a comprehensive review of controlled outcome research. *Psychol Bull.*, 108(1):30-49.

Rupke SJ, Blecke D, Renfrow M (2006). Cognitive therapy for depression. *Am Fam Phys.*, 73(1):83-6.

Rush AJ, Beck AT, Kovacs M, Hollon SD (1977). Comparative efficacy of cognitive therapy and pharmacotherapy in the treatment of depressed out-patients. *Cog Ther Res.*, 1:17-37.

Scher CD, Segal ZV, Ingram RE (2006). Beck's theory of depression: origins, empirical status, and future directions for cognitive vulnerability. In: Leahy RL, editor. *Contemporary cognitive therapy: theory, research, and practice*. New York: Guilford Press.

Sudak DM (2006). *Cognitive behavioral therapy for clinicians*. Philadelphia: Lippincott, Williams & Wilkins.

Teasdale JD, Moore RG, Hayhurst H, Pope M, Williams S, Segal ZV (2002). Metacognitive awareness and prevention of relapse in depression: empirical evidence. *J Consult Clin Psychol.*, 70(2):275-87.

Teasdale JD, Segal ZV, Williams JM, Ridgeway VA, Soulsby JM, Lau MA (2000). Prevention of relapse/recurrence in major depression by mindfulness- based cognitive therapy. *J Consult Clin Psychol.*, 68(4):615-23.

Thase ME (2006). Pharmacotherapy of bipolar depression: an update. *Curr Psychiatr Rep.,* 8:478-88.

Wexler BE, Cicchetti DV (1992). The outpatient treatment of depression. Implications of outcome research for clinical practice. *J Nerv Ment Dis.,* 180(5):277-86.

5

Cognitive Behavioral Therapy for Somatoform Disorders

Robert L. Woolfolk[1,2] and Lesley A. Allen[2,3]
[1]Rutgers University,
[2]Princeton University,
[3]UMDNJ – Robert Wood Johnson Medical School,
USA

1. Introduction

Somatoform disorders are characterized by physical symptoms that suggest a medical condition but that are not fully explained by a medical condition. Patients presenting with somatoform disorders represent a formidable challenge to the health care system. These patients tend to overuse health care services, derive little benefit from treatment, and experience protracted impairment, often lasting many years (Smith, Monson, & Ray, 1986a). Many patients with somatoform symptoms are dissatisfied with the medical services they receive and repeatedly change physicians (Lin et al., 1991). Likewise, physicians of these treatment-resistant patients often feel frustrated by patients' frequent complaints and dissatisfaction with treatment (Hahn, 2001; Lin et al., 1991). Because standard medical care has been relatively unsuccessful in treating somatoform disorders, alternative treatments have been developed. Cognitive-behavioral therapy (CBT) has been the most widely studied alternative treatment for these disorders.

Although medicine has long recognized a group of patients with medically unexplained physical symptoms, excessive health concerns, and abnormal illness behavior, there has been and continues to be disagreement over precise diagnostic labels and criteria. The history of the somatoform disorders begins with hysteria and hypochondriasis. The Egyptians were the first to describe hysteria about 4,000 years ago. Typical cases involved pain in the absence of any injury or pathology in the location of the pain. The Egyptian theory held that a wandering uterus moved about the body and produced pain from various regions (Veith, 1965). The Greeks gave us the word *hysteria*, from the Greek *hystera*, meaning womb. Hypochondriasis, also recognized in ancient times, was attributed to disturbances in the upper abdominal organs, such as the spleen and the stomach (Ladee, 1966).

The category of somatoform disorders was not officially recognized until the publication of DSM-III. The original DSM-III category of somatoform disorders included somatization disorder, hypochondriasis, conversion disorder, psychogenic pain disorder, and a residual somatoform disorder category (APA, 1980). The subsequent two editions of DSM included the same disorders with variations in their labels and diagnostic criteria (APA, 1987, 1994). Dysmorphophobia, later named body dysmorphic disorder, was considered a residual somatoform disorder in DSM-III and categorized as a distinct disorder in DSM-III-R and DSM-IV (APA, 1980, 1987, 1994). Table 1 outlines the disorders included in each of the editions of DSM.

The chapter provides a review of the diagnostic criteria for the somatoform disorders, according to DSM-IV. Also, summarized is the research on the demographic and clinical characteristics of patients who meet criteria for somatoform disorders as well as the randomized controlled trials examining the efficacy of cognitive behavioral therapy (CBT) for somatoform disorders. Future directions for classification and treatment are also discussed.

DSM-III	DSM-III-R	DSM-IV	Proposed DSM-5
Somatization disorder	Somatization disorder	Somatization disorder	
Hypochondriasis	Hypochondriasis	Hypochondriasis	Complex somatic symptom dis
Psychogenic pain disorder	Somatoform pain disorder	Pain disorder	Simple somatic symptom dis
	Undifferentiated somatoform disorder	Undifferentiated somatoform disorder	Illness anxiety disorder
Conversion disorder	Conversion disorder	Conversion disorder	Neurological functional disorder
Atypical somatoform disorder	Body dysmorphic disorder	Body dysmorphic disorder	
	Somatoform disorder NOS	Somatoform disorder NOS	
			Psychological factors affecting medical condition

Table 1. Somatoform Disorders 1980 - Present

2. Somatization disorder and subthreshold somatization

2.1 Diagnostic criteria and prevalence

In DSM-IV somatization disorder is characterized by a lifetime history of at least four unexplained pain complaints (e.g., in the back, chest, joints), two unexplained non-pain gastrointestinal complaints (e.g., nausea, bloating), one unexplained sexual symptom (e.g., sexual dysfunction, irregular menstruation), and one pseudo-neurological symptom (e.g., seizures, paralysis, numbness) (APA, 1994). For a symptom to be counted toward the diagnosis of somatization disorder its presence must be medically unexplained or its degree of severity be substantially in excess of the associated medical pathology. Also, each symptom must either prompt the seeking of medical care or interfere with the patient's functioning. In addition, at least some of the somatization symptoms must have occurred prior to the patient's 30th birthday (APA, 1994). The course of somatization disorder tends to be characterized by symptoms that wax and wane, remitting only to return later and/or be replaced by new unexplained physical symptoms. Thus, somatization disorder is a chronic, polysymptomatic disorder whose requisite symptoms need not be manifested concurrently.

Epidemiological research suggests that somatization disorder is relatively rare. The prevalence of somatization disorder in the general population has been estimated to be 0.1% to 0.7% (Faravelli et al., 1997; Robins & Reiger, 1991; Weissman, Myers, & Harding, 1978). When patients in primary care, specialty medical, and psychiatric settings are assessed, the rate of somatization is higher than in the general population, with estimates ranging from 1.0% to 5.0% (Altamura et al., 1998; Fabrega, Mezzich, Jacob, & Ulrich, 1988; Fink, Steen Hansen, & Søndergaard, 2005; Gureje, Simon, et al., 1997; Kirmayer & Robbins, 1991; Peveler, Kilkenny, & Kinmoh, 1997).

Although somatization disorder is classified as a distinct disorder in DSM-IV, it has been argued that somatization disorder represents the extreme end of a somatization continuum (Escobar, Burnam, Karno, Forsythe, & Golding, 1987; Kroenke, et al., 1997). The number of unexplained physical symptoms reported correlates positively with the patient's degree of emotional distress and functional impairment (Katon, et al., 1991). A broadening of the somatization construct has been advocated by those wishing to underscore the many patients encumbered by unexplained symptoms that are not numerous enough to meet criteria for full somatization disorder (Escobar, et al., 1987; Katon et al., 1991; Kroenke et al., 1997).

DSM-IV includes a residual diagnostic category for subthreshold somatization cases. *Undifferentiated somatoform disorder* is a diagnosis characterized by one or more medically unexplained physical symptom(s) that are distressing and/or disruptive and that have lasted for at least six months (APA, 1994). Long considered a category that is too broad because it includes patients with only one unexplained symptom as well as those with many unexplained symptoms, undifferentiated somatoform disorder never has been well-validated or widely applied (Kroenke, Sharpe, & Sykes, 2007).

Two research teams have suggested categories for subthreshold somatization using criteria less restrictive and requiring less extensive symptomatology than the standards for DSM-IV's full somatization disorder. Escobar and colleagues proposed the label, *abridged somatization*, to be applied to men experiencing four or more unexplained physical symptoms or to women experiencing six or more unexplained physical symptoms (Escobar, et al., 1987). Kroenke et al. suggested the category of *multisomatoform disorder* to describe men or women currently experiencing at least three unexplained physical symptoms and reporting a two-year history of somatization (Kroenke et al., 1997).

Both of these subthreshold somatization categories appear to be significantly more prevalent than is *somatization disorder* as defined by DSM-IV. Abridged somatization has been observed in 4% of community samples (Escobar, et al., 1987) and 16% to 22% of primary care samples (Escobar, Waitzkin, Silver, Gara, & Holman, 1998; Gureje, Simon et al., 1997; Kirmayer & Robbins, 1991). The occurrence of multisomatoform disorder has been estimated at 8% of primary care patients (Jackson & Kroenke, 2008; Kroenke et al., 1997).

2.2 Demographic and clinical characteristics

The demographic characteristic most often associated with somatization is gender. In the Epidemiological Catchment Area (ECA) study, women were 10 times more likely to meet criteria for somatization disorder than were men (Swartz, Landermann, George, Blazer, & Escobar, 1991). Higher rates of occurrence in women, though not as extreme, also have been found in most studies employing subthreshold somatization categories, such as Escobar's abridged somatization or Kroenke's multisomatoform disorder (Escobar, Rubio-Stipec, Canino, & Karno, 1989; Kroenke et al., 1997). A more complex picture of the association between gender and somatization was suggested by the WHO's Cross-National study in which female primary care patients were more likely to meet criteria for full somatization disorder, but no more likely to meet Escobar's abridged somatization criteria than were their male counterparts (Gureje, Simon, et al., 1997). On the severe end of the continuum, somatization disorder is uncommon in men. Gender differences are less obvious in the various subthreshold syndromes.

Ethnicity, race, and education have been associated with somatization disorder and subthreshold somatization. Epidemiological research has shown somatization patients more likely to be non-white and less educated than non-somatizers (Gureje, Simon, et al., 1997; Robins & Reiger, 1991). Findings on ethnicity have been less consistent across studies. In the ECA study, Hispanics were no more likely to meet criteria for somatization disorder than were non-Hispanics (Robins & Reiger, 1991). The WHO study, conducted in 14 different countries, revealed a higher incidence of somatization, as defined by either ICD-10 or Escobar's abridged criteria, in Latin American countries than in the United States (Gureje, Simon, et al., 1997).

Much attention has focused on somatization patients' illness behavior and the resulting impact of that behavior on the health care system. These patients disproportionately use and misuse health care services. When standard diagnostic evaluations fail to uncover organic pathology, somatization patients tend to seek additional medical procedures, often from several different physicians. Patients may even subject themselves to unnecessary hospitalizations and surgeries, which introduce the risk of iatrogenic illness (Fink, 1992). One study found that somatization disorder patients, on average, incurred nine times the US per capita health care cost (Smith et al., 1986a). Abridged somatization and multisomatoform disorder also have been associated with significant health care utilization (Barsky, Orav, & Bates, 2005; Escobar, Golding, Hough, Karno, Burnam, & Wells, 1987; Kroenke et al., 1997).

The abnormal illness behavior of somatizing patients extends beyond medical offices and hospitals to patients' workplaces and households. Somatizers withdraw from both productive and pleasurable activities because of discomfort, fatigue, and/or fears of exacerbating their symptoms. In a study assessing the efficacy of cognitive behavior therapy for somatization disorder, we found 19% of patients meeting DSM-IV criteria for somatization disorder to be receiving disability payments from either their employers or the government (Allen, Woolfolk, Escobar, Gara, & Hamer, 2006). Estimates of unemployment among somatization disorder patients range from 36% to 83% (Allen et al., 2006; Smith et al., 1986a; Yutzy et al., 1995). Whether working outside their homes or not, these patients report substantial functional impairment. Some investigators have found that somatization disorder patients report being bedridden for 2 to 7 days per month (Katon et al., 1991; Smith et al., 1986a). Likewise, high levels of functional impairment have been associated with subthreshold somatization (Allen, Gara, Escobar, Waitzkin, Cohen-Silver, 2001; Escobar, Golding, et al., 1987; Gureje, Simon, et al., 1997; Jackson & Kroenke, 2008; Kroenke et al., 1997).

In addition to their physical complaints, many somatization patients complain of psychiatric distress. As many as 80% of patients meeting criteria for somatization disorder or subthreshold somatization meet DSM criteria for another lifetime Axis I disorder, usually an anxiety or mood disorder (Smith et al., 1986a; Swartz, Blazer, George, & Landerman, 1986). When investigators consider only current psychiatric diagnoses, rates of Axis I psychiatric co-morbidity associated with somatization are closer to 50% (Allen, Gara, Escobar, Waitzkin, Cohen-Silver, 2001; Simon & Von Korff, 1991). Rates of Axis II psychiatric co-morbidity also are high (Garcia-Campayo, Alda, Sobradiel, Olivan, & Pascual, 2007; Rost, Akins, Brown, & Smith, 1992). Also, overall severity of psychological distress, defined as the number of psychological symptoms reported, correlates positively with the number of functional somatic symptoms reported (Katon et al., 1991; Simon & Von Korff, 1991).

2.3 Cognitive behavioral treatment

A number of studies have been conducted examining the efficacy of cognitive behavioral therapy (CBT) for somatization disorder or for subthreshold somatization. Two studies enrolled patients with at least one somatization symptom. Two other studies enrolled patients with multiple medically unexplained symptoms. Only study one enrolled patients meeting DSM-IV criteria for somatization disorder, the most severely disturbed somatizing patients. Various different approaches to integrating CBT into primary care have also been investigated.

The earliest randomized controlled trials on CBT for somatization included patients presenting with relatively mild levels of somatization, patients presenting with at least one psychosomatic symptom. The treatment protocols included identifying and restructuring dysfunctional cognitions, behavioral activation or reengaging patients in avoided activities, problem-solving, and relaxation training (Lidbeck, 1997; Speckens et al., 1995). In the first study patients treated with 6 to 16 sessions of individually-administered CBT showed significantly greater improvement in their psychosomatic complaints than did patients treated with standard medical care (Speckens et al., 1995). The other study found an 8-session group CBT superior to a waiting-list control condition in reducing physical symptoms and hypochondriacal beliefs (Lidbeck, 1997). In both studies improvements were observed after treatment as well as six months later (Lidbeck, 1997; Speckens et al., 1995). Both of these studies were conducted in primary care offices, the setting where somatization is most likely to be seen.

Two more recently published randomized controlled trials examined the efficacy of CBT for somatization with patients presenting with more severe somatization than the earlier trials. One study required participants meet Escobar's criteria of abridged somatization. That is, men were required to experience at least four somatization symptoms and women were required to experience at least six somatization symptoms (Escobar et al., 2007). The other trial enrolled participants who complained of five or more unexplained physical symptoms (Sumathipala, Hewege, Hanwella, & Mann, 2000). In both studies patients were identified and treated with CBT in primary care. Treatment protocols were similar to that of Lidbeck (1997) and Speckens et al., (1995) with the addition of involving the patient's spouse or other family member in treatment (Escobar et al., 2007; Sumathipala et al., 2000). Findings from both trials show individual CBT coincided with greater reductions in somatic complaints than did standard medical care (Escobar et al., 2007; Sumathipala et al., 2000). CBT was associated with a reduction in the number of physician visits in one study (Sumathipala et al., 2000).

We are the only group of researchers who have published a randomized controlled trial on the efficacy of CBT for full somatization disorder (Allen, Woolfolk, Escobar, Gara, & Hamer, 2006). In the study 84 patients meeting DSM-IV criteria for somatization disorder were randomly assigned to one of two conditions: (1) standard medical care or (2) a 10-session manualized individually-administered CBT in combination with standard medical care. The treatment protocol included relaxation training, activity regulation, facilitation of emotional awareness, cognitive restructuring, and interpersonal communication. Although the elicitation and exploration of affect is an approach rarely used in CBT, we have found this component to be a powerful clinical tool with patients who cannot or do not willingly access and experience emotion. We have described our treatment in detail elsewhere (Woolfolk & Allen, 2007). Participants' symptomatology and functioning were assessed with clinician-administered instruments, self-report questionnaires, and medical records before randomization as well as 3 months, 9 months, and 15 months after randomization. Just after the completion of treatment as well as one year later, i.e., at the 15-month follow-up assessment, patients who received CBT experienced a greater reduction in somatization and functional impairment. Substantially more participants who received CBT than the control treatment were rated as either "very much improved" or "much improved" by a clinician who was blind to participants' treatment condition (40% vs. 5%, respectively). Also, for the 68% of the sample for whom complete medical records were reviewed, CBT was associated with a reduction in health care costs and physician visits (Allen et al., 2006). Thus, the study suggests CBT can result in long-term improvements in the symptomatology, functioning, and health care utilization of the most severely disturbed somatizing patients.

2.4 Integrating CBT into primary care

Because somatization is so prevalent in primary care practices (Escobar, Waitzkin et al., 1998; Gureje, Simon et al., 1997; Kirmayer & Robbins, 1991), other approaches to the treatment of somatization have been focused on primary care physicians' behavior. Smith and colleagues sent a psychiatric consultation letter to patients' primary care physicians, describing somatization disorder and providing recommendations to guide primary care (Smith, Monson, & Ray, 1986b). The recommendations to physicians were straightforward: (a) to schedule somatizers' appointments every 4 to 6 weeks instead of "as needed", (b) to conduct a physical examination in the organ system or body part relevant to the presenting complaint, (c) to avoid diagnostic procedures and surgeries unless clearly indicated by underlying somatic pathology, and (d) to avoid making disparaging statements, such as "your symptoms are all in your head." Patients whose primary physicians had received the consultation letter experienced better health outcomes, such as physical functioning and cost of medical care, than those whose physicians had not received the letter. The results were replicated in three additional studies, one study using patients meeting criteria for full somatization disorder (Rost, Kashner, & Smith, 1994) and two studies using patients with subthreshold somatization (Dickinson, et al., 2003; Smith, Rost, & Kashner, 1995).

Given the success of the above-described consultation letter and the success of CBT, some investigators have attempted to train primary care physicians to better detect somatization and to incorporate cognitive and behavioral techniques into their treatment of these patients. Five groups of investigators have reported controlled clinical trials on the effects of such physician training (Arnold et al., 2009; Larish, Schweickhardt, Wirsching, & Fritzsche, 2004; Morriss et al., 2007; Rief, Martin, Rauh, Zech, & Bender, 2006; Rosendal et al., 2007). The two studies providing the most extensive physician training (20-25 hours) resulted in no association between physician training and patients' symptomatology, functioning, or quality of life (Arnold et al., 2009; Rosendal et al., 2007). Three other studies found less intensive physician training programs, 12 hours (Larish et al., 2004) or 1 day (Rief et al., 2006) or six hours (Morriss et al., 2007) to coincide with no clear improvement in somatization symptomatology; however, Rief and colleagues did find their training to coincide with fewer health care visits for the 6 months subsequent to training (Rief et al., 2006).

One other study examined the effect of training primary care clinicians to identify and treat somatization using a biopsychosocial model (Smith et al., 2006). This study involved the most intensive such training programs studied, one entailing 84 hours over 10 weeks. Nurse practitioners were trained to provide a year-long 12-session multidimensional intervention in primary care that incorporated biopsychosocial conceptualizations of, behavioral recommendations for, and medication management of somatization. Patients who received treatment from these trained nurses reported modest improvements on self-report scales of mental health such as mood and energy and physical functioning. A post hoc analysis was interpreted by the study's investigators as suggesting improvements were attributable to more frequent and appropriate use of antidepressant medication among patients of nurses who received the training (Smith et al., 2006).

A slightly different model for integrating CBT into primary care is a collaborative care model of treatment, in which mental health professionals work together with medical practitioners in the primary care setting (Katon et al., 1995; von Korff, Gruman, Schaefer, Curry & Wagner, 1997). The one study investigating the efficacy of such a model for the treatment of somatization had psychiatrists provide primary care physicians and their staff with training on the diagnosis and treatment of somatization and comorbid psychopathology (van der Feltz-Cornelis, van Oppen, Ader, & van Dyck, 2006). Also, the psychiatrist provided case-specific consultations to primary physicians regarding referrals for CBT and/or psychiatric treatment (van der Feltz-Cornelis et al., 2006). A control comparison treatment included the same training for primary care physicians and their staff by the psychiatrist without the case-specific consultation. Six months after randomization, participants whose primary care physician received psychiatric consultation reported a greater reduction in somatic symptoms and in health care visits (van der Feltz-Cornelis et al., 2006).

In all, the literature on the treatment of somatization supports the use of 6-16 sessions of CBT administered by a mental health professional. A recent meta-analysis indicated CBT is modestly effective in reducing somatization symptomatology and minimally effective improving physical functioning (Kleinstäuber, Witthöft, & Hiller, 2011). To date there is no evidence that CBT reduces health care services when the cost of CBT itself is considered. Researchers have just begun to develop and examine the effectiveness of true collaboration between cognitive behavioral therapists and primary care clinicians and integration of their services.

3. Hypochondriasis

3.1 Diagnostic criteria and prevalence

According to DSM-IV, hypochondriasis is defined as a "preoccupation with fears of having, or the idea that one has, a serious disease based on the person's misinterpretation of bodily symptoms" (APA, 1994, p. 462). This preoccupation must last for at least six months, persist despite medical evaluation and physician reassurance, and cause significant distress or impairment in one's functioning (APA, 1994). Thus, unlike in somatization where the distress and dysfunction experienced is due to the physical symptoms themselves, in hypochondriasis the distress and dysfunction is due to the patient's interpretation of the meaning of his or her symptoms. The course of hypochondriasis is often chronic: As many as 50% of patients meeting DSM criteria for hypochondriasis have excessive health concerns for many years (Barsky, Fama, Bailey & Ahern, 1998; Barsky, Wyshak, Klerman, & Latham, 1990).

There are only a few epidemiological studies that have examined the prevalence of hypochondriasis. Studies that have utilized a clinical interview to assess prevalence have suggested that hypochondriasis occurs rarely in the general population. Such estimates range from 0.02 to 1.6% (Faravelli et al., 1997; Looper & Kirmayer, 2001; Martin & Jacobi, 2006). In primary care, estimates range from 0.8% to 6.3% (Barsky et al., 1990; Escobar, Gara, et al. 1998; Gureje, Ustun, & Simon, 1997).

3.2 Demographic and clinical characteristics

Unlike somatization disorder, hypochondriasis does not appear to be related to gender (Barsky et al, 1990; Gureje, et al., 1997; Looper & Kirmayer, 2001). Men are as likely to meet DSM criteria for hypochondriasis as are women. Findings have been inconsistent on whether hypochondriasis is related to education, socio-economic status, and ethnicity (Barsky et al., 1990; Gureje, et al., 1997).

Like patients with somatization disorder and milder versions of somatization disorder, those with hypochondriasis exhibit abnormal illness behavior. They over-utilize health care (Gureje, Ustun, et al., 1997; Looper & Kirmayer, 2001), subjecting themselves to multiple physician visits and multiple diagnostic procedures. They report great dissatisfaction with their medical care (Barksy, 1996; Noyes et al., 1993). In addition, patients diagnosed with hypochondriasis report substantial physical impairment and functional limitations related to employment (Escobar et al., 1998; Gureje, Ustun, et al., 1997; Looper & Kirmayer, 2001; Noyes et al., 1993). Also, hypochondriasis frequently co-occurs with other Axis I disorders, such as mood, anxiety, or other somatoform disorders (Gureje, Ustun, et al., 1997; Noyes et al., 1994) and various Axis II disorders (Sakai, Nestoriuc, Nolido, & Barsky, 2010).

3.3 Cognitive behavioral treatment

Psychosocial treatments for hypochondriasis have been examined in six randomized controlled trials. The interventions in all six studies were brief (i.e., 6 to 16 sessions), theoretically grounded in social learning theory, and administered on an individual basis. Three groups of investigators examined the efficacy of CBT (Barsky & Ahern, 2004; Greeven et al., 2007; Warwick, Clark, Cobb, & Salkovskis, 1996). Two other trials examined the efficacy of treatments, labeled cognitive therapy (CT) (Clark et al., 1998; Visser & Bouman, 2001). Behavioral stress management, exposure in vivo plus response prevention, and explanatory therapy have also been studied, each in one randomized controlled trial. Below we provide an elaboration of the specific interventions and a review of the studies' findings.

All treatments labeled CBT or CT involved identifying and challenging patients' misinterpretations of physical symptoms as well as constructing more realistic interpretations of them (Barsky & Ahern, 2004; Clark et al., 1998; Greeven et al., 2007; Visser & Bouman, 2001; Warwick, Clark, Cobb, & Salkovskis, 1996). Visser and Bouman's (2001) CT consisted of a "pure CT" that focused on only cognitive elements of treatment. Clark et al.'s CT (1998), on the other hand appears to be procedurally similar to the point of being indistinguishable from many of those labeled CBT for hypochondriasis (Greeven et al., 2007; Warwick, Clark, Cobb, & Salkovskis, 1996). Specifically, most CBT and Clark et al.'s CT combined cognitive restructuring with exposure to interoceptive and/or external stimuli along with response prevention after exposure (Clark et al., 1998; Greeven et al., 2007; Warwick et al., 1996). Barsky and Ahern's CBT did not include exposure plus response prevention. Instead, they attempted to reduce patients' tendency to amplify physical symptoms and to alter patients' illness behaviors, in addition to restructuring cognitions (Barsky & Ahern, 2004). Another difference among the treatments was their durations. Barsky and Ahern's (2004) treatment entailed six 90-min sessions. Visser and Bouman's (2001) intervention consisted of 12 weekly sessions, each presumably lasting 1 hour, though session duration was not indicated. The duration of Greeven et al.'s (2007) CBT which was "based on the treatment protocol used by Visser and Bouman," (p. 93) ranged from 6 to 16 sessions. Both Clark et al.'s (1998) and Warwick et al.'s (1996) treatments involved 16 1-hour sessions.

All CT and CBT interventions were associated with significantly greater reductions in hypochondriacal symptoms than was the comparable waiting list or standard medical care control condition (Barsky & Ahern, 2004; Clark et al., 1998; Greeven et al., 2007; Visser & Bouman, 2001; Warwick, et al., 1996). Barsky and Ahern's study was the only one that examined long-term differences between the control group and the treated group: Ten months after treatment completion, patients enrolled in CBT reported a greater decline in hypochondriacal cognitions than did controls. Also, Barsky and Ahren's CBT-treated participants reported a significantly greater increase in daily activities than did controls, even 10 months after treatment (Barsky & Ahern, 2004).

In addition to their pure CT condition, Visser and Bouman (2001) also assessed the efficacy of a largely behavioral intervention, exposure plus response prevention. Patients receiving this treatment constructed hierarchies of their own hypochondriacal fears and avoidance behavior patterns, such as checking, reassurance seeking, avoidance of interoceptive and/or external stimuli. Afterwards, they were given assignments of in vivo exposure and response prevention. Patients treated with exposure reported significantly greater reductions in their hypochondriacal symptoms than did wait-list control participants. Although Visser and Bouman also compared exposure plus response prevention to their CT intervention described above, the study was not sufficiently powerful to distinguish between the two treatments.

Clark et al. (1998) created a psychosocial alternative to CT, behavioral stress management (BSM) that did not directly address hypochondriacal concerns. It was intended to address anxiety related to hypochondriasis by training patients in relaxation, problem-solving, assertiveness training, and time management. Clark et al. (1998) found behavioral stress management significantly more effective in alleviating hypochondriacal concerns than was a waiting list. Clark et al. also compared this treatment to their CT described earlier. At post-treatment CT-treated participants experienced greater reductions in their hypochondrical cognitions than did BSM-treated participants. Nevertheless, 12 months after the post-treatment assessment, these differences were not observed (Clark et al., 1998).

Finally, Fava et al. examined the efficacy of explanatory therapy (Kellner, 1983) for hypochondriasis, in hopes of identifying a beneficial treatment that is less complex and easier to administer than CBT (Fava, Grandi, Rafanelli, Fabbri, & Cazzaro, 2000). Explanatory therapy is a physician-administered individual therapy consisting of patient education, reassurance, and training in selective attention (i.e., reducing somatic attention). Like the cognitive and behavioral treatments described above, explanatory therapy resulted in greater reductions in worry about illness than did the waiting list (Fava et al., 2000). Although explanatory therapy was also associated with greater reductions in physician visits than was the control group, the mean reduction in visits was minimal (3 visits) considering the treatment group received 8 additional visits as part of their explanatory therapy (Fava et al., 2000).

The one study comparing a psychosocial intervention with a pharmacological intervention demonstrated that CBT was more effective than a placebo pill, but no more effective than paroxetine, in reducing hypochondriacal beliefs (Greeven et al., 2007). Despite the statistical significance of these findings, the clinical significance of changes observed in this study suggests that patients experienced only modest improvement. Instead of using Jacobson's recommendation of a change of 1.96 standard deviations from the pretreatment mean as an index of clinically significant change, the investigators judged as clinically significant a change of 1.0 standard deviation. Using this more lenient criterion, only 45% of CBT recipients and 30% of paroxetine recipients versus 14% of waiting list controls responded to treatment at clinically significant levels (Greeven et al. 2007).

3.4 Integrating CBT into primary care

Given the prevalence of hypochondriasis in medical practices (Barsky et al., 1990; Escobar, Gara, et al., 1998; Gureje, Ustun, et al., 1997), it would seem important to develop treatments to be administered in medical settings. Only one of the randomized controlled trials described above was conducted in primary care (Barsky & Ahern, 2004). All other trials were conducted in mental health or psychosomatic medicine clinics, and thus leave open to question the generalizability of findings to hypochondriacal primary care patients. Will primary care patients with concerns about their physical health be open to a treatment designed to challenge the validity of those concerns? A significant proportion (29%) of the patients recruited for Barsky and Ahern's study declined to participate (Barsky & Ahern, 2004). Future research could examine the efficacy of CBT that is integrated and coordinated with primary care.

4. Conversion disorder

4.1 Diagnostic criteria and prevalence

Conversion symptoms, also described as pseudo-neurological symptoms, are abnormalities or deficits in voluntary motor or sensory function that are medically unexplained. Some of the most common pseudo-neurological symptoms are pseudo-seizures, pseudo-paralysis and psychogenic movement disorders. According to DSM-IV, conversion disorder is characterized by the presence of one or more pseudo-neurological symptoms that are distressing and/or disruptive and are associated with psychological stressor(s) or conflict(s). Also, the symptoms can not be intentionally produced or feigned (APA, 1994). The diagnosis of conversion disorder requires a thorough psychiatric evaluation as well as a physical examination in order to rule out organic neurological illness. Patients presenting with conversion symptoms typically have normal reflexes and normal muscle tone.

The course of conversion disorder appears to be different from that of somatization disorder, which tends to be chronic (Kent, Tomasson, & Coryell, 1995). The onset and course of conversion disorder often take the form of an acute episode. Symptoms may remit within a few weeks of an initial episode and they may recur in the future. Some research indicates that a brief duration of symptoms prior to treatment is associated a better prognosis (Crimlisk et al., 1998; Hafeiz, 1980; Ron, 2001).

Estimates of the prevalence of conversion disorder have varied widely, ranging from 0.01 to 0.3% in the community (Faravelli et al., 1997; Stefansson, Messina, & Meyerowitz, 1979). As is the case with the other somatoform disorders, conversion disorder is much more common in medical and psychiatric practices than in community samples. As many as 25% of neurology clinic patients may present for treatment of a medically unexplained neurological symptom (Creed, Firth, Timol, Metcalf & Pollock, 1990; Perkin, 1989).

4.2 Demographic and clinical characteristics

The demographic characteristics of conversion disorder have not been investigated extensively. Nevertheless, there is some evidence that conversion disorder is more common among women (Deveci et al., 2007; Faravelli et al., 1997), non-whites (Stefansson, et al., 1979), and individuals from lower socioeconomic classes (Folks, Ford, & Regan, 1984; Stefansson, et al., 1979). Co-morbid psychiatric distress in patients with pseudo-neurological symptoms is high; it has been estimated that 30% to 90% of patients seeking treatment for pseudo-neurological symptoms also meet criteria for at least one other psychiatric disorder, typically somatoform disorders, affective disorders, anxiety disorders, or personality disorders (Binzer, Andersen, & Kullgren, 1997; Crimlisk et al., 1998; Mokleby, Akyuz, Kundakel, Kizitlan & Dogan, 2002; Sar et al., 2004). A co-morbid personality disorder diagnosis has been found to indicate poor prognosis of conversion disorder (Mace & Trimble, 1996).

Like somatization disorder, conversion disorder is costly to the health care system, especially when symptoms are chronic (Mace & Trimble, 1996). Patients with long-standing conversion symptoms are likely to submit themselves to unnecessary diagnostic and medical procedures. Martin and colleagues reported an average of $100,000 being spent per year per conversion disorder patient (Martin, Bell, Hermann, & Mennemeyer, 2003).

4.3 Cognitive behavioral treatment

We are aware of only one published randomized controlled trial investigating the efficacy of CBT for conversion disorder. In the study patients diagnosed by a neurologist as having psychogenic nonepileptic seizures were randomly assigned to receive standard neuropsychiatry care alone or standard neuropsychiatry care plus individual CBT (Goldstein et al., 2010). The 12-session CBT was designed to help patients interrupt behavioral, physiological, and emotional responses that occurred at the onset of seizures. Specifically, patients were encouraged to engage in avoided activities, utilize relaxation methods, and restructure their dysfunctional cognitions (Goldstein et al., 2010). At the conclusion of treatment, patients who received CBT reported a greater reduction in psychogenic seizures than did the control group. At the 6-month follow up assessment, the difference between treatment and control groups was only marginally significant. Health care utilization and social and work functioning did not change differentially between the treatment groups (Goldstein et al., 2010).

5. Pain disorder

5.1 Diagnostic criteria and prevalence

Pain disorder is characterized by clinically significant pain that is judged to be affected by psychological factors (APA, 1994). Very little research has been conducted that addresses pain disorder as defined by DSM-IV (or its counterparts, psychogenic pain disorder and somatoform pain disorder in DSM-III and DSM-III-R, respectively) as a discrete diagnostic category. Instead, researchers have tended to formulate research based on the anatomical site and the chronicity of the pain. Thus, there is a voluminous literature on distinct pain conditions, e.g., back pain, chest pain, pelvic pain, headaches. In very few of these studies have investigators attempted to distinguish between pain that was apparently affected by psychological factors and pain that was apparently not, presumably because such a distinction is too difficult to make and perhaps unreliable.

The few investigators who have examined the epidemiology of somatoform pain disorder, instead of specific pain syndromes, have not assessed whether psychological factors were involved in the onset, severity, exacerbation, or maintenance of the pain, as required by DSM-IV. Instead, the diagnosis was made for medically unexplained pain that lasted six months and impaired functioning. In these studies, somatoform pain disorder had a one-year prevalence of 0.6% to 8.1% (Faravelli et al., 1997; Frohlich, Jacobi, & Wittchen, 2005) and a lifetime prevalence of 12.3% (Grabe et al., 2003).

Given the difficulty of determining whether psychological factors are associated pain symptoms and the similarity of the presentation of pain disorder with that of somatization disorder and subthreshold somatization, many experts have suggested the elimination of the pain disorder category from future versions of DSM (Birket-Smith & Mortenson, 2002; Kroenke, et al., 2007; Sullivan, 2000). In fact, the most recent proposal for DSM-5 has eliminated this diagnostic label (APA, 2010).

5.2 Demographic and clinical characteristics

The limited body of research on pain disorder suggests that it is associated with functional impairment, overuse of medical services, and psychopathology (Frohlich et al., 2005).

5.3 Cognitive behavioral treatment

We are not aware of any published randomized controlled trial investigating the efficacy of CBT for DSM-IV pain disorder or for the DSM-III or DSM-III-R counterparts to it. Reviews on CBT for specific pain disorders, such as non-cardiac chest pain, chronic back pain, headaches, can be found elsewhere and are consistent with the findings for other somatoform disorders showing CBT to be associated with modest benefits in symptomatology (Kisely, Campbell, Skerritt, & Yelland, 2010; Kröner-Herwig, 2009).

6. Body dysmorphic disorder

6.1 Diagnostic criteria and prevalence

DSM-IV body dysmorphic disorder (BDD) is characterized by a preoccupation with an imagined defect in appearance. If a slight physical irregularity is present, the person's concern must be excessive to be meet criteria for BDD. Also required for a diagnosis of BDD is significant distress or impairment caused by this preoccupation (APA, 1994). Typically, patients are concerned about their skin or complexion, the size of the nose or head, or the attractiveness of the hair; however, the preoccupation may concern any body part.

BDD tends to be chronic. In one study Phillips at al. found only a 0.09 probability of full remission and 0.21 probably of partial remission over the course of a year (Phillips, Pagano, Menard, & Stout, 2006).

The prevalence of BDD is uncertain. Research conducted in community settings has produced varying estimates: a prevalence of 0.7% in a community setting in Italy (Faravelli et al., 1997), 1.7 % in a national survey of German adolescents and adults (Reif, Buhlmann, Wilhelm, Borkenhagen, & Brähler, 2006), and 2.4% in a telephone survey of U.S. adults (Koran, Abujaoude, Large, & Serpe, 2008). The prevalence of BDD in medical practices has been found to be substantially higher than that found in the general population: 4% of general medicine patients (Phillips, 1996), 3% to 16% of cosmetic surgery patients (Sarwer & Crerand, 2008), and 8% to 15% of dermatology patients (Sarwer & Crerand, 2008).

6.2 Demographic and clinical characteristics

Relatively little research has been conducted on sex and cultural differences in BDD. Two groups of investigators have found that women and men were equally likely to meet criteria for BDD (Koran, Abujaoude, Large & Serpe, 2008; Phillips & Diaz, 1997). We are aware of no systematic investigation of race and culture in BDD, though the condition has been described in various cultures around the world (Phillips, 1996).

Patients meeting criteria for BDD have been shown to have substantial functional impairment (Phillips, 2000). Negative thoughts about one's appearance interfere with concentration at work and the social lives of patients. In addition, individuals with BDD are so afraid of exposing their flaw to others that they go to great lengths to hide it. They may spend substantial amounts of time camouflaging their perceived defect or avoiding activities in which they will be conspicuous (Phillips, McElroy, Keck, Pope, & Hudson, 1993). Avoidance of social activities and work is common (Phillips et al., 1993).

Health care use associated with BDD tends to be directed toward seeking various appearance enhancing medical treatments, especially cosmetic surgery and dermatological procedures. For patients with BDD these treatments typically fail to alleviate distress (Crerand, et al., 2005; Phillips, Grant, Siniscalchi, & Albertini, 2001). Investigators have found that 48% to 76% of patients with BDD sought cosmetic surgery, dermatological treatment, or dental procedures (Crerand, et al., 2005; Phillips, et al., 2001; Veale, Boocock, et al., 1996) and 26% received multiple procedures (Veale, Boocock, et al., 1996).

Patients meeting criteria for BDD experience an enormous amount of emotional distress and psychiatric co-morbidity (Phillips, Menard, Fay, & Weisberg, 2005; Veale, Boocock, et al., 1996). Depression and suicidal thoughts are frequent (Gunstad & Phillips, 2003; Phillips & Menard, 2006). Also common is social phobia and obsessive compulsive disorder (Gunstad & Phillips, 2003). Often, compulsions are related to the perceived physical defect, such as checking mirrors or brushing one's hair. Many of these patients also admit to substance, particularly alcohol, use and dependence disorders (Grant, Menard, Pagano, Fay, & Phillips, 2005; Gunstad & Phillips, 2003). Co-morbid personality disorders are likely to be present (Phillips & McElroy, 2000).

Many patients preoccupied with an imagined defect in their physical appearance have such inaccurate perceptions of their appearance that they meet DSM-IV criteria for delusional disorder, somatic type. About 50% of clinical samples meeting criteria for BDD also meet criteria for delusional disorder, somatic type (Phillips, McElroy, & Keck, 1994); however, instead of considering this somatic type of delusional disorder a co-morbid condition with BDD, a growing body of research suggests psychotic variants of BDD are simply more severe forms of non-psychotic BDD and are, therefore, best conceived as on the same continuum. It seems that non-psychotic and psychotic BDD share the same demographic characteristics, clinical characteristics, and response to treatment (Phillips, 2004). Further evidence suggests that the cognitions of BDD patients involving such matters as the degree of conviction with which they hold their beliefs are more indicative of a dimensional rather than a categorical structure (Phillips, 2004). Thus, the research data suggest a dimensional model of BDD with varying levels of insight indicating severity of the condition.

6.3 Cognitive behavioral treatment

Only two randomized controlled trials have been published on the efficacy of CBT for BDD (Rosen, Reiter, & Orosan, 1995; Veale, Gournay, et al., 1996). Both interventions involved the restructuring dysfunctional beliefs about one's body and exposure to avoided situations plus response prevention, for example, preventing checking behavior and reassurance seeking. Whereas Rosen et al.'s treatment was administered in eight 2-hour group sessions, Veale et al. administered treatment in 12 weekly individual sessions. Both groups of investigators compared the effects of CBT with those of a waiting list control condition.

Both studies provided strong evidence for the short-term efficacy of CBT for BDD. Rosen et al. found that 81.5% of treated participants but only 7.4% of control participants experienced clinically significant improvement, in that their scores on the Body Dysmorphic Disorder Examination (BDDE) dropped more than two standard deviations *and* they no longer met criteria for BDD. The effect size on the BDDE was substantial (d = 2.81) (Rosen et al., 1995). Follow-up assessment, occurring 4.5 months after post-treatment, was conducted with only CBT participants, 74% of whom continued to have achieved clinically meaningful gains (Rosen et al., 1995). Veale et al. reported that at post-treatment 77.8% of the treatment group either had absent or sub-clinical BDD symptomatology whereas all waiting list participants still met criteria for BDD. Furthermore, Veale's effect size on the BDDE and on a BDD-modified Yale Brown Obsessive Compulsive Scale were also noteworthy (d = 2.65 and 1.81, respectively) (Veale, Gournay, et al., 1996). Follow-up was not investigated in this study.

In all, CBT for BDD must be considered an evidence based treatment. Although the potency of the treatments described in these two well-designed controlled trials is noteworthy, a number of questions remain about the efficacy of CBT for BDD. No additional randomized controlled trials have been published. CBT has not been compared with alternative treatments nor with an attention control. It is unclear whether treatment gains reported above could be attributable to nonspecific aspects of therapy. Also, long-term follow-up has not been adequately studied. Other important outcomes, such as physical and social functioning and health care use, have not been assessed. Finally, the generalizability of these findings is unclear. Between the two studies only 36 patients have been treated. Rosen et al.'s sample consisted of women, 83% of whom had body weight and shape concerns. Veale et al.'s sample specifically excluded potential participants with body weight and shape concerns.

6.4 Integrating CBT into primary care

Given that patients with BDD are likely to seek treatment from medical practitioners, treatment should be administered in primary care. Also, primary care physicians are likely to require training in identifying BDD. No published study has assessed an attempt to integrate CBT into primary care.

7. Future research

7.1 Future research on the classification of somatoform disorders

In the midst of much debate over nosology of the somatoform disorders (Hyler & Spitzer, 1978; Mayou, Kirmayer, Simon, Kroenke, & Sharpe, 2005), a number of changes have been proposed for DSM-5 by the DSM-5 Somatic Symptom Disorders Work Group (APA, 2010). As a general framework for these disorders, there is a shift from emphasizing the functional-status of somatic symptoms (i.e., that symptoms be medically unexplained) to the dysfunctional thoughts, feelings and behaviors related to somatic symptoms. The mind-body dualism implied by the construct of medically unexplained symptoms as well as the unreliability of assessments of a symptom's true cause (e.g., organic vs. functional) have long been identified as shortcomings (Jablensky, 1999; Mayou et al., 2005). Also, numerous clinician-researchers have expressed concern using pejorative labels (Kirmayer, 1988). In line with these concerns, the terms somatoform, somatization, and hypochondriasis have been eliminated from the most recent proposal for DSM-5 (APA, 2010). The overall category will be renamed, somatic symptom disorders. Detailed below are the most recent proposals for changes to the specific diagnostic categories within somatic symptom disorders group, that is, the creation of diagnostic categories and removal of others.

7.1.1 Complex somatic symptom disorder

A new category, complex somatic symptom disorder, has been proposed to subsume somatization disorder, undifferentiated somatoform disorder, somatoform pain disorder, and most cases of hypochondriasis. The rationale for grouping together these disorders is that their "similarities outweigh their differences" (Dimsdale et al., 2009). As is demonstrated in this chapter, a review of the research from the past 30 years indicates the clinical characteristics of patients meeting criteria for somatization disorder, undifferentiated somatoform disorder, pain disorder, and hypochondriasis (i.e., their presentation of somatic symptoms, incorrect illness attributions, health anxiety, and abnormal illness behavior) are almost identical. In reviewing the epidemiology of somatization disorder and hypochondriasis, Creed and Barksy state there is not sufficient evidence to distinguish between even these two disorders (Creed & Barsky, 2004). The similarity in treatment response also has been used to argue for a combining of these categories (Dimsdale et al., 2009). In addition, the DSM-5 Somatic Symptom Disorders Work Group cite the research showing physicians see the somatoform disorders as overlapping disorders (Dimsdale, Sharma, & Sharpe, 2011) as a rationale for uniting somatization disorder, undifferentiated somatoform disorder, pain disorder and hypochondriasis (APA, 2010).

To receive a diagnosis of complex somatic symptom disorder, patients must complain of at least one somatic symptom that is distressing and/or disruptive of their daily lives. Also, patients must have at least two of the following emotional/cognitive/behavioral disturbances: high levels of health anxiety, disproportionate and persistent concerns about the medical seriousness of the symptom(s), and an excessive amount of time and energy devoted to the symptoms and health concerns. Finally, the symptoms and related concerns must have lasted for at least six months.

Future research will examine the epidemiology, clinical characteristics, or treatment of complex somatic symptom disorder as there is no published research on this diagnostic category.

7.1.2 Simple somatic symptom disorder

Also new to DSM-5 is the category, simple somatic symptom disorder, which will be used to classify somatically-focused presentations that are more transient and presumably less severe than those meeting criteria for complex somatic symptom disorder. Specifically, simple somatic symptom disorder will be characterized by somatic concerns that have lasted for at least one month and that are accompanied by at least one of the emotional/cognitive/behavioral disturbances listed in the previous section (e.g., health anxiety, concerns about medical seriousness of symptom, or abnormal illness behavior) (APA, 2010). Just as for complex somatic symptom disorder, there is no published research on the epidemiology, clinical characteristics, or treatment of simple somatic symptom disorder.

7.1.3 Illness anxiety disorder

Although the DSM-5 Somatic Symptom Disorders Work Group states that most cases of DSM-IV hypochondriasis are likely to meet criteria for DSM-5 complex somatic symptom disorder (APA, 2010), an additional category has been created for patients whose health anxiety is not associated with any somatic symptoms. This new category, illness anxiety disorder, will be characterized by the presentation of *no* somatic symptoms, or only those mild in severity, and a preoccupation with having or acquiring a serious illness. Also required for the diagnosis are significant health anxiety about having or acquiring a serious illness, excessive behaviors to check one's illness status or maladaptive behaviors to avoid illness concerns, and a persistence of the illness concerns for at least six months (APA, 2010). We are not aware of any published research on the epidemiology, clinical characteristics, or treatment response of patients presenting with this "pure" form illness anxiety.

7.1.4 Functional neurological disorder

The proposal for conversion disorder in DSM-5 is to retain the category with slight changes. First, the category will be renamed functional neurological disorder. Second, DSM-IV's requirement that the symptom(s) not be intentionally produced or feigned by the patient will be eliminated, given the difficulty clinicians are likely to have making such a determination. Also no longer required will be the judgment that psychological factors are associated with the symptom(s). Functional neurological disorder is the one somatic symptom disorder category that will retain the dualistic diagnostic criterion of the symptom(s) being medically unexplained. The DSM-5 Somatic Symptom Disorders Work Group cites the recent evidence that neurologists can reliably make the distinction between organic and functional neurological symptoms (Stone, 2009).

7.1.5 Other disorders

The current plan for BDD is to move it from the somatic symptom disorders section to the obsessive-compulsive and related disorders section (APA, 2010). The research showing the similarities between the symptomatology and treatment response of BDD and obsessive-compulsive disorder (Castle, Rossell, & Kyrios, 2006) has been used to justify this change. The diagnostic criteria for DSM-5 BDD now specify that patients need to have performed repetitive behaviors or mental acts in response to appearance concerns at some point during the disorder (APA, 2010).

A new addition to the somatic symptom disorders group will psychological factors affecting medical condition that has resided in the "other conditions" category. This regrouping has been suggested because this condition, whose diagnostic criteria appear to have minimal change from that in DSM-IV, is characterized by the presentation of somatic symptoms and/or distress regarding a medical condition (APA, 2010). Specifically, the DSM-5 criteria include (1) the presence of a general medical condition, (2) psychological or behavioral factors that affect the medical condition. Again, this change is consistent with the attempt to avoid distinguishing between medically explained and unexplained physical symptoms.

7.2 Future research on cognitive behavioral treatment of somatoform disorders

One hurdle in administering CBT to somatically-focused patients is that most of these patients seek treatment in primary care, not in psychiatric clinics. When patients with somatoform symptoms are referred to mental health treatment, it is estimated that 50 to 90% of these patients fail to complete the referral (Escobar, Waitzkin, et al., 1998; Reiger et al.,

1988). Impediments to successful psychiatric referral of patients presenting with somatization occur at both the professional institutional level (e.g., lack of collaboration between primary care and mental health practitioners, lack of mental health training for primary care physicians, inadequate mental health insurance) and level of the individual patient (e.g., concerns about the stigma of having a psychiatric disorder, resistance to psychiatric diagnosis, health beliefs that lead to somatic presentations, pessimism, and fatigue) (Freidl et al., 2007; Pincus, 2003). This literature suggests that the effectiveness of CBT for the somatoform disorders would be enhanced if treatment were conducted in primary care settings where the overwhelming majority of these patients are seen. Also, as suggested by the research on somatization, an integration of mental health providers into primary care and collaboration with primary care physicians and staff would seem imperative in that it could increase the acceptability and availability of CBT. Additional research is required to substantiate these recommendations.

As we move forward to refine the treatment of patients with somatic symptom disorders, one direction for future research is to improve treatment outcome. As a whole, cognitive and behavioral treatments have been shown to reduce physical discomfort, health anxiety, and functional limitations in these patients. Although even the most severely and chronically disturbed somatization and hypochondriacal patients have benefited from treatment, a majority of the treated patients continued to suffer with significant symptomatology after treatment ended (see Woolfolk & Allen, 2007, for review). Long-term benefits have been demonstrated in only a few trials. Also, there is little data on the impact of treatment on health care utilization, especially when the cost of a psychosocial intervention is factored in to the equation. The investigation of longer-term treatments has been recommended for patients who are severely or chronically disturbed (Woolfolk & Allen, 2007). Some researchers have argued for studying a stepped-care approach in which all patients would receive low-intensity targeted primary care management. Response to this initial phase of treatment would guide the level of intensity of additional treatment and possible referral to mental health specialists (Arnold et al., 2009; Fink & Rosendal, 2008).

We have very little data on the mechanisms by which cognitive behavioral treatments have their impact upon somatoform disorders. There are multiple reasons for this. First, the mediators and moderators style of research has not been extensively applied to research on somatoform disorders. Second, the treatments studied have not been disassembled into discrete components and those constituents systematically assessed. Evidence that might shed some light on this issue, that pertaining to differential efficacy of treatment, is also scant. This absence of evidence, to some extent, is the result of much overlap among treatments. When reading the somatoform treatment literature, careful attention must be paid to methods sections, as the labeling of treatments can often be somewhat misleading. Future research could be directed towards examining what components of CBT are most beneficial to somatic symptoms vs. cognitive dysfunctions vs. health anxiety vs. abnormal illness behavior.

8. Conclusion

Although the literature on the specific somatoform disorders is relatively small, a few global conclusions can be posited. CBT for somatization, hypochondriasis, and BDD has been empirically supported. Specific elements of the cognitive behavioral interventions examined for the different somatoform disorders are outlined in Table 2. There is inadequate data on the treatment of conversion disorder or of pain disorder to make any conclusion.

Diagnosis	Elements of CBT
Somatization disorder/Undifferentiated somatoform disorder	Identifying and restructuring cognitions Altering illness behavior/Behavioral activation Relaxation training Involvement of spouse or family member Elicitation and expression of emotion
Hypochondriasis	Identifying and restructuring cognitions Exposure plus response prevention
Conversion Disorder	Identifying and restructuring cognitions Altering illness behavior/behavioral activation Relaxation training
Body dysmorphic disorder	Identifying and restructuring cognitions Exposure plus response prevention
Pain disorder	--

Table 2. Specific elements of CBT examined with specific somatoform disorders

An evaluation of the empirical research on CBT for somatoform disorders suggests that in some respects it mirrors the literature on evaluating the efficacy of psychotherapy literature with various mental disorders. CBT has been shown to be superior to various control conditions, especially waiting lists or standard medical treatment. Effect sizes are respectable, relative to other medical or quasi-medical interventions.

There are three clear directions recommended for enhancing the efficacy and effectiveness of CBT for somatoform disorders. The first is to treat patients in the treatment setting where they seek treatment, i.e., primary care settings. Second is to integrate mental health care providers into the primary care treatment setting. And, the third is to increase the length of CBT for patients who are willing to engage in CBT. Two meta-analyses, one on psychosocial treatments of somatization (Kleinstäuber, Witthöft, & Hiller, 2011), the other on psychosocial treatment of hypochondriasis (Thomson & Page, 2007), found a positive association between length of treatment and outcome, suggesting longer term treatments may be more potent.

The treatment of somatoform disorders via CBT is very much in its infancy. The methodological quality of the early research has been uneven. Nevertheless, there is sufficient evidence to believe that cognitive behavioral interventions have therapeutic value for a number of the disorders. For somatization, hypochondriasis, and BDD, CBT is the treatment of choice given that no other intervention has demonstrated efficacy.

9. References

Allen, L. A., Escobar, J. I., Lehrer, P. M., Gara, M. A., & Woolfolk, R. L. (2002). Psychosocial treatments for multiple unexplained physical symptoms: A review of the literature. Psychosomatic Medicine, 64, 939-950.

Allen, L. A., Gara, M. A., Escobar, J. I., Waitzkin, H., & Cohen-Silver, R. (2001). Somatization: A debilitating syndrome in primary care. Psychosomatics, 42, 63-67.

Allen, L. A., Woolfolk, R. L., Escobar, J. I., Gara, M. A., & Hamer, R. M. (2006). Cognitive-behavioral therapy for somatization disorder: A randomized controlled trial. Archives of Internal Medicine, 166, 1512-1518.

Altamura, A. C., Carta, M. G., Tacchini, G., Musazzi, A., Pioli, M. R., & the Italian Collaborative Group on Somatoform Disorders. (1998). Prevalence of somatoform disorders in a psychiatric population: An Italian nationwide survey. European Archives of Psychiatry and Clinical Neuroscience, 248, 267-271.

American Psychiatric Association. (1980). Diagnostic and statistical manual of mental disorders (3rded.). Washington, DC: Author.

American Psychiatric Association. (1987). Diagnostic and statistical manual of mental disorders (3rd ed., rev.). Washington, DC: Author.

American Psychiatric Association. (1994). Diagnostic and statistical manual of mental disorders (4th ed.). Washington, DC: Author.

American Psychiatric Association. (2010). DSM-5 Development. Available at: http://www.dsm5.org/proposedrevision/Pages/SomaticSymptomDisorders.aspx Accessed August 15, 2011.

Arnold, I. A., de Waal, M. W., Eekhof, J. A., Assendelft, W. J., Spinhoven, P., van Hemert, A. M. (2009). Medically unexplained physical symptoms in primary care: A controlled study on the effectiveness of cognitive-behavioral treatment by the family physician. Psychosomatics, 50, 515-524.

Barsky, A. J., & Ahern, D. K. (2004). Cognitive behavior therapy for hypochondriasis: A randomized controlled trial. Journal of the American Medical Association, 291, 1464-1470.

Barsky, A. J., Fama, J. M., Bailey, E., D., & Ahern, D. K. (1998). A prospective 4- to 5-year study of DSM-III-hypochondriasis. Archives of General Psychiatry, 55, 737-744.

Barsky, A. J., Orav, E. J., & Bates, D. W. (2005). Somatization increases medical utilization and cost independent of psychiatric and medical utilization. Archives of General Psychiatry, 62, 903-910.

Barsky, A. J., Wyshak, G., Klerman, G. L., & Latham, K. S. (1990). The prevalence of hypochondriasis in medical outpatients. Social Psychiatry and Psychiatric Epidemiology, 25, 89-94.

Binzer, M., Andersen, P. M., & Kullgren, G. (1997). Clinical characteristics of patients with motor disability due to conversion disorder: A prospective control group study. Journal of Neurology Neurosurgery and Psychiatry, 63, 83–88.

Birket-Smith, M., & Mortensen, E. L. (2002). Pain in somatoform disorders: Is somatoform pain disorder a valid diagnosis? Acta Psychiatrica Scandanavica, 106, 103-108.

Castle, D. J., Rossell, S., & Kyrois, M. (2006). Body dysmorphic disorder. Psychiatric Clinics of North America, 29, 521-538.

Chambless, D. L., & Hollon, S. D. (1998). Defining empirically supported therapies. Journal of Consulting and Clinical Psychology, 66, 7-18.

Clark, D. M., Salkovskis, P. M., Hackmann, A., Wells, A., Fennell, M., Ludgate, J., Ahmad, S., Richards, H. C., & Gelder, M. (1998). Two psychological treatments for hypochondriasis: A randomised controlled trial. British Journal of Psychiatry, 173, 218-225.

Creed, F., & Barksy, A. J. (2004). A systematic review of somatisation and hypochondriasis. Journal of Psychosomatic Research, 56, 391-408.

Creed, F., Firth, D., Timol, M., Metcalfe, R., & Pollock, S. (1990). Somatization and illness behaviour in a neurology ward. Journal of Psychosomatic Research, 34, 427–437.

Crerand, C. E., Phillips, K. A., Menard, W., & Fay, C. (2005). Nonpsychiatric medical treatment of body dysmorphic disorder. Psychosomatics, 46, 549-555.

Crimlisk, H. L., Bhatia, K., Cope, H., David, A., Marsden, C. D., Ron, M. A. (1998). Slater revisited: 6-year follow-up study of patients with medically unexplained motor symptoms. British Medical Journal, 316, 582-586.

Deveci, A., Taskin, O., Dinc, G., Yilmaz, H., Demet, M. M., Erbay-Dundar, P., Kaya, E., & Ozmen, E. (2007). Prevalence of pseudoneurological conversion disorder in an urban community in Manisa, Turkey. Social Psychiatry and Psychiatric Epidemiology, 42, 857-864.

Dickinson, W. P., Dickinson, L. M., deGruy, F. V., Main, D. S., Candib, L. M., & Rost, K. (2003). A randomized clinical trial of a care recommendation letter intervention for somatization in primary care. Annals of Family Medicine, 1, 228-235.

Dimsdale, J., Creed, F. & the work group. (2009). The proposed diagnosis of somatic symptom disorders in DSM-5 to replace somatoform disorders in DSM-IV: A preliminary report. Journal of Psychosomatic Research, 66, 473-476.

Dimsdale, J., Sharma, N., & Sharpe, M. (2011). What do physicians think of somatoform disorders. Psychosomatics, 52, 154-159.

Escobar, J. I., Burnam, A., Karno, M., Forsythe, A., & Golding J. M. (1987). Somatization in the community. Archives of General Psychiatry, 44, 713-718.

Escobar, J. I., Gara, M. I., Diaz-Martinez, A. M., Interian, A., Warman, M., Allen, L. A., Woolfolk, R. L., Jahn, E., Rodgers, D. (2007). Effectiveness of a time-limited cognitive behavior therapy–type intervention among primary care patients with medically unexplained symptoms. Annals of Family Medicine, 5, 328-335.

Escobar, J. I., Gara, M., Waitzkin, H., Silver, R. C., Holman, A., & Compton, W. (1998). DSM-IV hypochondriasis in primary care. General Hospital Psychiatry, 20, 155-159.

Escobar, J. I., Golding, J. M., Hough, R. L., Karno, M., Burnam, M. A., & Wells, K. B. (1987). Somatization in the community: Relationship to disability and use of services. American Journal of Public Health, 77, 837-840.

Escobar, J. I., Rubio-Stipec, M., Canino, G., & Karno, M. (1989). Somatic symptom index (SSI): A new and abridged Somatization construct. Prevalence and epidemiological correlates in two large community samples. Journal of Nervous and Mental Disease, 177, 140-146.

Escobar, J. I., Waitzkin, H., Silver, R. C., Gara, M., & Holman, A. (1998). Abridged somatization: A study in primary care. Psychosomatic Medicine, 60, 466-472.

Fabrega, H., Mezzich, J., Jacob, R., & Ulrich, R. (1988). Somatoform disorder in a psychiatric setting: Systematic comparisons with depression and anxiety disorders. Journal of Nervous and Mental Disease, 176, 431-439.

Faravelli, C., Salvatori, S., Galassi, F., Aiazzi, L., Drei, C., & Cabras, P. (1997). Epidemiology of somatoform disorders: A community survey in Florence. Social Psychiatry and Psychiatric Epidemiology, 32, 24-29.

Fava, G. A., Grandi, S., Rafanelli, C., Fabbri, S., & Cazzaro, M. (2000). Explanatory therapy in hypochondriasis. Journal of Clinical Psychiatry, 61, 317-322.

Fink, P. (1992). Surgery and medical treatment in persistent somatizing patients. Journal of Psychosomatic Research, 36, 439-447.

Fink, P., & Rosendal, M. (2008). Recent developments in the understanding and management of functional somatic symptoms in primary care. Current Opinion in Psychiatry, 21, 182-188.

Fink, P., Steen Hansen, M., & Søndergaard, L. (2005). Somatoform disorders among first-time referrals to a neurology service. Psychosomatics, 46, 540-548.

Folks, D. G., Ford, C. V., & Regan, W. M. (1984). Conversion symptoms in a general hospital. Psychosomatics, 25, 285-295.

Freidl, M., Spitzl, S. P., Prause, W., Zimprich, F., Lehner-Baumgartner, E., Baumgartner, C., & Aigner, M. (2007). The stigma of mental illness: Anticipation and attitudes among patients with epileptic, dissociative or somatoform pain disorder. International Review of Psychiatry, 19, 123–129.

Frohlich, C., Jacobi, F., & Wittchen, H. U. (2005). DSM-IV pain disorder in the general population. A exploration of the structure and threshold of medically unexplained pain symptoms. European Archives of Psychiatry and Clinical Neuroscience, 256 187-196.

Garcia-Campayo, J., Alda, M., Sobradiel, N., Olivan, B., & Pascual, A. (2007). Personality disorders in somatization disorder patients: A controlled study in Spain. Journal of Psychosomatic Research, 62, 675-680.

Goldstein, L. H., Chalder, T., Chigwedere, C., Khondoker, M. R., Moriarty, J., Toone, B. K., & Mellers, J. D. (2010). Cognitive-behavioral therapy for psychogenic nonepileptic seizures: A pilot RCT. Neurology, 74, 1986-1994.

Grabe, H. J., Meyer, C., Hapke, U., Rumpf, H. J., Frevberger, H. J., Diling, H., & John, U. (2003). Somatoform pain disorder in the general population. Psychotherapy and Psychosomatics, 72, 88-94.

Grant, J. E., Menard, W., Pagano, M. E., Fay, C. & Phillips, K. A. (2005). Substance use disorders in individuals with body dysmorphic disorder. Journal of Clinical Psychiatry, 66, 309-316.

Greeven A., van Balkom, A. J., Visser, S., Merkelbach, J. W., vanRood, Y. R., van Dyck, R., Van der Does, A. J., Zitman, G. F., & Spinhoven, P. (2007). Cognitive behavior therapy and paroxetine in the treatment of hypochondriasis: A randomized controlled trial. American Journal of Psychiatry, 164, 91-9.

Gunstad, J. & Phillips, K. A. (2003). Axis I comorbidity in body dysmorphic disorder. Comprehensive Psychiatry, 44, 270- 276.

Gureje, O., Simon, G. E., Ustun, T., Goldberg, D. P. (1997). Somatization in cross-cultural perspective: A World Health Organization study in primary care. American Journal of Psychiatry, 154, 989-995.

Gureje, O., Ustun, T. G., & Simon, G. E. (1997). The syndrome of hypochondriasis: A cross-national study in primary care. Psychological Medicine, 27, 1001-1010.

Hafeiz, H. B. (1980). Hysterical conversion: A prognostic study. British Journal of Psychiatry, 136, 548-551.

Hahn, S. R. (2001). Physical symptoms and physician-experienced difficulty in the physician-patient relationship. Annals of Internal Medicine, 134, 897-904.

Hyler, S. E., & Spitzer, R. L. (1978). Hysteria aplit asunder. American Journal of Psychiatry, 135, 1500-1504.

Jablensky, A. (1999). The concept of somatoform disorders: A comment on the mind-body problem in psychiatry. In Y. Ono, A. Janca, M. Asai, & N. Sartorius (Eds.), Somatoform Disorders: A Worldwide Perspective (pp. 3-10). New York: Springer-Verlag.

Jackson, J. L., & Kroenke, K. (2008). Prevalence, impact, and prognosis of multisomatoform disorder in primary care: A 5- year follow-up study. Psychosomatic Medicine, 70, 430-434.

Katon, W., Lin, E., Von Korff, M., Russo, J., Lipscomb, P., & Bush, T. (1991). Somatization: A spectrum of severity. American Journal of Psychiatry, 148, 34-40.

Kellner, R. (1983). Prognosis of treated hypochondriasis. Acta Psychiatrica Scandanavica, 67, 69-76.

Kent, D. A., Tomasson, K., Coryell, W. (1995). Course and outcome of conversion and somatization disorder. A four-year follow-up. Psychosomatics, 36, 138-144.

Kirmayer, L. J. (1988). Mind and body as metaphors: Hidden values in biomedicine. In M. J. Lock, D. R. Gordon (Eds.), Biomedicine Examined (pp. 57-93). Boston, MA: Kluwer.

Kirmayer, L. J., & Robbins, J. M. (1991). Three forms of somatization in primary care: Prevalence, co-occurrence, and sociodemographic characteristics. Journal of Nervous and Mental Disease, 179, 647-655.

Kisely, S., Campbell, L. A., Skerritt, P., & Yelland, M. J. (2010). Psychological interventions for symptomatic management of non-specific chest pain in patients with normal coronary anatomy. Cochrane Database of Systematic Reviews, 1. CD004101.

Koran, L. M., Abujaoude, E., Large, M.D., & Serpe, R. T. (2008). The prevalence of body dysmorphic disorder in the United States adult population. CNS Spectrums, 13, 316-322.

Kroenke, K. (2007). Efficacy of treatment for somatoform disorders. A review of randomized controlled trials. Psychosomatic Medicine, 69, 881-889.

Kroenke, K., Sharpe, M., & Sykes, R. (2007). Revising the classification of somatoform disorders: Key questions and preliminary recommendations. Psychosomatics, 48, 277-285.

Kroenke, K., Spitzer, R. L., deGruy, F. V., Hahn, S. R., Linzer, M., Williams, J. B., Brody, D., & Davies, M. (1997). Multisomatoform disorder: An alternative to undifferentiated somatoform disorder for the somatizing patient in primary care. Archives of General Psychiatry, 54, 352-358.

Kröner-Herwig, B. (2009). Chronic pain syndromes and their treatment by psychological interventions. Current Opinion in Psychiatry, 22, 200-204.

Ladee, G. A. (1996). Hypochondriacal Syndromes. Amerstam, The Netherlands: Elsevier.

Larisch, A., Schweickhardt, A., Wirsching, M., & Fritzsche, K. (2004). Psychosocial interventions for somatizing patients by the general practitioner: A randomized controlled trial. Journal of Psychosomatic Research, 57, 507–514.

Lidbeck, J. (1997). Group therapy for somatization disorders in general practice: Effectiveness of a short cognitive- behavioural treatment model. Acta Psychiatrica Scandinavica, 96, 14-24.

Lin, E. H., Katon, W., Von Korff, M., Bush, T., Lipscomb, R., Russo, J., & Wagner, E. (1991). Frustrating patients: Physician and patient perspectives among distressed high users of medical services. Journal of General Internal Medicine, 6, 241-246.

Looper, K. J., & Kirmayer, L. J. (2001). Hypochondriacal conerns in a community population. Psychological Medicine, 31, 577-584.

Katon, W., von Korff, M., Lin, E., Walker, E., Simon, G. E., Bush, T., Robinson, P., & Russo, J. (1995). Collaborative management to achieve treatment guidelines. Impact on depression in primary care. Journal of the American Medical Association, 273, 1026-1031.

Kleinstäuber, M., Witthöft, M., & Hiller, W. (2011). Efficacy of short-term psychotherapy for multiple medically unexplained physical symptoms: A meta-analysis. Clinical Psychology Review, 31, 146-160.

Mace, C. J., & Trimble, M. R. (1996). Ten-year prognosis of conversion disorder. British Journal of Psychiatry, 169, 282-288.

Martin, A., & Jacobi, F. (2006). Features of hypochondriasis and illness worry in the general population in Germany. Psychosomatic Medicine, 68, 770-777.

Martin, R., Bell, B., Hermann, B., & Mennemeyer, S. (2003). Non epileptic seizures and their costs: The role of neuropsychology. In G. P. Pritigano & N. H. Pliskin (Eds.), Clinical Neuropsychology and Cost Outcome Research: A beginning (pp. 235-258). New York: Psychology Press.

Mayou, R., Kirmayer, L. J., Simon, G., Kroenke, K., & Sharpe, M. (2005). Somatoform disorders: Time for a new approach in DSM-V. American Journal of Psychiatry, 162, 847-855.

Mokleby, K., Blomhoff, S., Malt, U. F., Dahlström, A., Tauböll, E., & Gjerstad, L. (2002). Psychiatric comorbidity and hostility in patients with psychogenic nonepileptic seizures compared with somatoform disorders and healthy controls. Epilepsia, 43, 193–198.

Morriss, R., Dowrick, C., Salmon, P., Peters, S., Dunn, G., Rogers, A., Lewis, B., Charles-Jones, H., Hogg, J., Clifford, R., Rigby, C., & Gask, L. (2007). Cluster randomised controlled trial of training practices in reattribution for medically unexplained symptoms. British Journal of Psychiatry, 191, 536-542.

Noyes, R., Kathol, R. G., Fisher, M. M., Phillips, B. M., Suelzer, M. T., & Holt, C. S. (1993).The validity of DSM-III-R hypochondriasis. Archives of General Psychiatry, 50, 961-970.

Noyes, R., Kathol, R. G., Fisher, M. M., Phillips, B. M., Suelzer, M. T., & Woodman, C. K. (1994). Psychiatric comorbidity among patients with hypochondriasis. General Hospital Psychiatry, 16, 78-87.

Parsons, T. (1951). Illness and the role of the physician: A sociological perspective. American Journal of Orthopsychiatry, 21, 452-460.

Perkin, G. D. (1989). An analysis of 7,836 successive new outpatient referrals. Journal of Neurology, Neurosurgery, and Psychiatry, 52, 447–448.

Peveler, R., Kilkenny, L., & Kinmonth A. L. (1997). Medically unexplained physical symptoms in primary care: A comparison of self-report screening questionnaires and clinical opinion. Journal of Psychosomatic Research, 42, 245-252.

Phillips, K. A. (1996). The broken mirror: Understanding and treating body dysmorphic disorder. New York, NY: Oxford University Press.

Phillips, K. A. (2000). Quality of life for patients with body dysmorphic disorder. Journal of Nervous and Mental Disease, 188, 170–175.

Phillips, K. A. (2004). Psychosis in body dysmorphic disorder. Journal of Psychiatric Research, 38, 63–72.

Phillips, K. A., & Diaz, S. (1997). Gender differences in body dysmorphic disorder. Journal of Nervous and Mental Disease, 185, 570–577.

Phillips, K. A., Grant, J., Siniscalchi, J., & Albertini, R. S. (2001). Surgical and nonpsychiatric medical treatment of patients with body dysmorphic disorder. Psychosomatics, 42, 504-510.

Phillips, K. A., & McElroy, S. L. (2000). Personality disorders and traits in patients with body dysmorphic disorder. Comprehensive Psychiatry, 41, 229-236.

Phillips, K. A., McElroy, S. L., & Keck, P. E. Jr. (1994). A comparison of delusional and nondelusional body dysmorphic disorder in 100 cases. Psychopharmacological Bulletin, 30, 179–186.

Phillips, K. A., McElroy, S. L., Keck, P. E. Jr., Pope, H. G. Jr., & Hudson, J. I. (1993). Body dysmorphic disorder: 30 cases of imagined ugliness. American Journal of Psychiatry, 150, 302-308.

Phillips, K. A., & Menard, W. (2006). Suicidality in body dysmorphic disorder: A prospective study. American Journal of Psychiatry, 163, 1280-1282.

Phillips, K. A., Menard, W., Fay, C., & Weisberg, R. (2005). Demographic characteristics, phenomenology, comorbidity, and family history in 200 individuals with body dysmorphic disorder. Psychosomatics, 46, 317-325.

Phillips, K. A., Pagano, M. E., Menard, W., & Stout, R. L. (2006). A 12-month follow-up study of the course of body dysmorphic disorder. American Journal of Psychiatry, 163, 907-912.

Pincus, H. A. (2003). The future of behavioral health and primary care: Drowning in the mainstream or left on the bank? Psychosomatics, 44, 1-11.

Reiger, D., Boyd, J., Burke, J., Rae, D. S., Myers, J. K., Kramer, M., Robins, L. N., George, L. K., Karno, M., Locke, B. Z. (1988). One-month prevalence of mental disorders in the US: based on five epidemiological catchment area sites. Archives of General Psychiatry, 45, 977-986.

Rief, W., Buhlmann, U., Wilhelm, S., Borkenhagen, A., & Brähler, E. (2006). The prevalence of body dysmorphic disorder: A population-based survey. Psychological Medicine, 36, 877-885.

Rief, W., Hessel, A., Braehler, E. (2001). Somatization symptoms and hypochondriacal features in the general population. Psychosomatic Medicine, 63, 595-602.

Rief, W., Hiller, W., & Margraf, J. (1998). Cognitive aspects of hypochondriasis and the somatization syndrome. Journal of Abnormal Psychology, 107, 587-595.

Rief, W., Martin, A., Rauh, E., Zech, T., & Bender, A. (2006). Evaluation of general practitioners' training: How to manage patients with unexplained physical symptoms. Psychosomatics, 47, 304 -311.

Ron, M. (2001). The prognosis of hysteria/somatization disorder. Contemporary approaches to the study of hysteria. Oxford: Oxford University Press.

Robins, L. N., & Reiger, D. (1991). Psychiatric disorders in America: The epidemiological catchment area study: New York: Free Press.

Rosen, J. C., Reiter, J., & Orosan, P. (1995). Cognitive-behavioral body image therapy for body dysmorphic disorder. Journal of Consulting and Clinical Psychology, 63, 263 - 269.

Rosendal, M., Olesen, F., Fink, P., Toft, T., Sokolowski, I., & Bro, F. (2007). A randomized controlled trial of brief training in the assessment and treatment of somatization in primary care: Effects on patient outcome. General Hospital Psychiatry, 29, 364 -373.

Rost, K. M., Akins, R. N., Brown, F. W., & Smith, G. R. (1992). The comorbidity of DSM-III-R personality disorders in somatization disorder. General Hospital Psychiatry, 14, 322-326.

Rost, K., Kashner, T. M., & Smith, G. R. (1994). Effectiveness of psychiatric intervention with somatization disorder patients: Improved outcomes at reduced costs. General Hospital Psychiatry, 16, 381-387.

Sakai, R., Nestoriuc, Y., Nolido, N. V., & Barsky, A. J. (2010). The prevalence of personality disorders in hypochondriasis. Journal of Clinical Psychiatry, 71, 41-47.

Sar, V., Akyuz, G., Kundakci, T., Kiziltan, E., & Dogan, O. (2004). Childhood trauma, dissociation, and psychiatric comorbidity in patients with conversion disorder. American Journal of Psychiatry, 161, 2271-2276.

Sarwer, D. B., & Crerand, C. E. (2008). Body dysmorphic disorder and appearance enhancing medical treatments. Body Image, 5, 50-58.

Simon, G. E., & VonKorff, M. (1991). Somatization and psychiatric disorder in the NIMH Epidemiologic Catchment Area Study. American Journal of Psychiatry, 148, 1494-1500.

Smith, G. R., Monson, R. A., Ray, D. C. (1986a). Patients with multiple unexplained symptoms: Their characteristics, functional health, and health care utilization. Archives of Internal Medicine, 146, 69-72.

Smith, G. R., Monson, R. A., & Ray, D. C. (1986b). Psychiatric consultation letter in somatization disorder. New England Journal of Medicine, 314, 1407-1413.

Smith, G. R., Rost, K., & Kashner, M. (1995). A trial of the effect of a standardized psychiatric consultation on health   outcomes and costs in somatizing patients. Archives of General Psychiatry, 52, 238-243.

Smith, R. C., Lyles, J. S., Gardiner, J. C., Sirbu, C., Hodges, A., Collins, C., Dwamena, F. C., Lein, C., Given, W. C., Given, B., & Goddeeris, J. (2006). Primary care clinicians treat patients with medically unexplained symptoms: A randomized controlled trial. Journal of General Internal Medicine, 21, 671–677.

Speckens, A. E. M., van Hemert, A. M., Spinhoven, P., Hawton, K. E., Bolk, J. H., & Rooijmans, G. M. (1995a). Cognitive behavioural therapy for medically unexplained physical symptoms: A randomised controlled trial. British Medical Journal, 311, 1328-1332.

Stefansson, J. G., Messina, J. A., & Meyerowitz, S. (1979). Hysterical neurosis, conversion type: Clinical and epidemiological considerations. Acta Psychiatrica Scandanavica, 53, 119-138.

Stone, J., Carson, A., Duncan, R., Coleman, R., Roberts, R., Warlow, C., Hibberd, C., Murray, G., Cull, R., Pelosi, A., Cavanagh, J., Matthews, K., Goldbeck, R., Smyth, R., Walker, J., Macmahon, A. D., & Sharpe M. (2009). Symptoms 'unexplained by organic disease' in 1144 new neurology out-patients: How often does the diagnosis change at follow-up? Brain, 132, 2878-2888.

Sullivan, M. D. (2000). DSM-IV Pain Disorder: A case against the diagnosis. International Review of Psychiatry, 12, 91-98.

Sumathipala, A., Hewege, S., Hanwella, R., & Mann, A. H. (2000). Randomized controlled trial of cognitive behaviour therapy for repeated consultations for medically unexplained complaints: A feasibility study in Sri Lanka. Psychological Medicine, 30, 747-757.

Swartz, M., Blazer, D., George, L., & Landerman, R. (1986). Somatization disorder in a community population. American Journal of Psychiatry, 143, 1403-1408.

Swartz, M., Landermann, R., George, L., Blazer, D., & Escobar, J. (1991). Somatization. In L. N. Robins & D. Reiger (Eds.), Psychiatric disorders in America (pp. 220-257). New York: Free Press.

Van der Feltz-Cornelis, C. M., van Oppen, P., Ader, H. J., & van Dyck, R. (2006). Randomised controlled trial of a collaborative care model with psychiatric consultation for persistent medically unexplained symptoms in general practice. Psychotherapy and Psychosomatics, 75, 282-289.

Veale, D., Boocock, A., Goumay, E., Dryden, W., Shah, R., Willson, R. & Walburn, J. (1996). Body dysmorphic disorder. A survey of fifty cases. British Journal of Psychiatry, 169, 196-201.

Veale, D., Gournay, K., Dryden, W., Boocock, A., Shah, F., Willson, R., & Walburn, J. (1996). Body dysmorphic disorder: A cognitive behavioural model and pilot randomised controlled trial. Behaviour Research and Therapy, 34, 717 - 729.

Veith, I. (1965). Hysteria: The History of a Disease. Chicago, IL: University of Chicago Press.

Visser, S., & Bouman, T. K. (2001). The treatment of hypochondriasis: Exposure plus response prevention vs. cognitive therapy. Behaviour Research and Therapy, 39, 423-442.

Von Korff, M., Gruman, J., Schaefer, J., Curry, S. J., Wagner, E. H. (1997). Collaborative management of chronic illness. Annals of Internal Medicine, 127, 1097-1102.

Warwick, H. M. C., Clark, D. M., Cobb, A. M., & Salkovskis, P. M. (1996). A controlled trial of cognitive-behavioural treatment of hypochondriasis. British Journal of Psychiatry, 169, 189-195.

Weissman, M. M., Myers, J. K., & Harding, P. S. (1978). Psychiatric disorders in a U.S. urban community: 1975-1976. American Journal of Psychiatry, 135, 459-462.

Woolfolk, R. L. & Allen, L. A. (2007). Treating Somatization: A Cognitive-Behavioral Approach. New York: Guilford Press.

Yutzy, S. H., Cloninger, R., Guze, S. B., Pribor, E. F., Martin, R. L., Kathol, R. G., Smith G. R., & Strain J. J. (1995). DSM-IV field trial: Testing a new proposal for somatization disorder. American Journal of Psychiatry, 152, 97-101.

6

Cognitive-Behavioral Therapy for the Bipolar Disorder Patients

Mario Francisco P. Juruena[1,2]
[1]Department of Neurosciences and Behaviour,
Faculty of Medicine Ribeirao Preto, University of Sao Paulo,
[2]Department Psychological Medicine, Institute of Psychiatry, King's College London
[1]Brazil
[2]U.K.

"When you are high, it is tremendous. Shyness goes, the right words and gestures are suddenly there, the power to seduce and captivate others a felt certainty. Feelings of ease, intensity, power, well-being, financial omnipotence and euphoria now pervade one's marrow. But somehow, this changes. The fast ideas are far too fast and there are far too many, overwhelming confusion replaced by fear and concern. You are irritable, angry, frightened, uncontrollable, and enmeshed totally in the blackest caves of mind… It goes on and on and finally there are only other people's recollections of your behaviour – your bizarre, frenetic, aimless behaviour…"
A patient's account from Goodwin & Jamison (1990)

1. Introduction

This chapter reviews cognitive therapy (CT) for bipolar disorder (BD). The poor outcome of patients diagnosed with BD supports the addition of a psychosocial intervention for the treatment of this recurring disorder. The psychoeducational nature of CT, the effectiveness in increasing compliance to pharmacological treatment and the ability to prevent relapse in unipolar depression are used in the treatment of mania and BD. Results indicate that CT may be an effective intervention for the treatment of BD. Specifically CT may be useful in improving quality of life and functioning, increasing compliance, helping early symptom recognition, decrease relapse and decrease depressive and maniac symptomatology. Understanding the cognitive process in BD can refine our cognitive interventions in BD.

This discussion is best initiated by considering some of the limitations of somatic treatment. Despite the significant pharmacopeia for bipolar disorder, the most common outcome continues to be a clinical course characterized by repeated episodes. For example, despite the use of mood-stabilizing agents, longitudinal data suggests relapse rates as high as 40% in 1 year, 60% in 2 years, and 73% in 5 or more years (Gitlin et al., 1995; see also O'Connell et al., 1991). Resolution of bipolar depression is also characterized by poor outcomes for patients despite the regular application of mood stabilizers (Keck et al., 1998), and overall, adherence to medication treatment brings with it its own challenges, with poor medication compliance evident in one-half to two-thirds of patients within the first 12 months of treatment (Keck et al., 1998, Keck et al., 1996). All of these findings encourage the search for additional modalities of intervention for bipolar disorder.

Between 1960 and 1998, there were over 30 published outcome studies describing the combined use of psychological and pharmacological treatments in BP. However, the majority were small scale, with an average sample size of about 25, giving a total sample for all studies was just over 1000 participants.

The majority of the papers addressed group (n=14) or family approaches (n=13), with only four papers reporting on individual therapy. Most importantly, about 20 of the studies were open cohort studies with no control treatment to compare with the experimental psychotherapy.

Although the studies also had many methodological limitations, it was clear in many of these studies that those receiving adjunctive psychological treatments had better subjective clinical and social outcomes than those receiving usual treatments (comprising mainly of mood stabilizers and outpatient support), and there was some evidence of observer-rated differences that reached statistical significance. These encouraging results facilitated the development of randomized controlled trials of more targeted interventions that have now been tested in more sophisticated randomized treatment trials.

The occurrence of negative life events has also been found to influence the course of recovery from episodes in patients with bipolar disorder. For example, in a study of 67 patients recruited during hospitalization for mania or depression, negative life events were associated with a threefold increase in time to recovery (Johnson and Miller, 1997). Similar effects were evident in a study of relapse prevention. Ellicott et al. (1990) found that rates of relapse were 4.5 times higher among patients with high negative life-event scores during a 2-year follow-up study.

Cognitive style also appears to play an important role in modulating the impact of life events on symptoms. For example, in combination with negative life stressors, bipolar individuals with dysfunctional attitudes or depressogenic attributional styles are more likely to develop affective symptoms (Alloy et al., 1999). These findings support the rationale for utilizing cognitive-behavioral interventions aimed at modifying maladaptive cognitive styles and decreasing the impact of environmental stress.

In the last 5 years, interest in psychosocial interventions in BP has increased dramatically with about 20 randomized controlled trials underway in the USA, UK and Europe. Given the current emphasis on the use of brief evidence-based therapies in clinical guidelines for the treatment of unipolar disorders, it is not surprising that the new treatment trials for BP have focused on psychoeducational models, the three most well-researched manualized psychological approaches: interpersonal social rhythms therapy (IPSRT), cognitive therapy (CT) and family focused therapy (FFT), or techniques derived directly from these manualized therapies. The latter are used primarily to improve illness awareness, medication adherence, to teach recognition of prodromes and relapse prevention techniques. Eight of the completed studies have produced data that can be included in a systematic review of relapse rates and allow a meta-analysis of relapse rates for adjunctive psychological treatments compared to usual psychiatric treatment (either routine or standardized).

The first five studies (Lam et al., 2000; Perry et al., 1999; Scott et al., 2001; Frank et al., 1999) were relatively small scale and used a variety of approaches, but predominantly focused on either cognitive behaviour therapy (CBT) or cognitive and behavioural techniques, or interpersonal social rhythms therapy (IPSRT). These RCTs, which used either treatment as usual or treatment as usual plus support or symptom management sessions as the control condition, demonstrated that psychological treatments appear to have some benefit in preventing relapse, but that the effect was more impressive for total relapses or depressive relapses rather than manic relapses.

The three largest studies published in the literature used either CBT (Lam et al., 2003), Family Therapy (Miklowitz et al., 2003) or Group Psycho-Education (Colom et al., 2003). A separate meta-analysis of outcome data from these RCTs using fixed and random effects models demonstrate that the odds ratio for relapse in the active as compared to the control treatment groups is similar to that reported for the earlier studies. There appear to be some differences in ORs between studies, but these may relate to sample characteristics (e.g. proportion of participants who met criteria for BP I or BP II) as well as similarities or differences in the style and content of the treatments. Importantly, the interventions all have a significant effect on rates of depressive relapses as well as reducing the frequency of manic episodes. So perhaps the treatment of syndromal and sub-syndromal depressive symptoms of BP might be improved by the use of these more complex and more extended interventions.

The basic aims of therapy in bipolar disorder (BP) are to alleviate acute symptoms, restore psychosocial functioning, and prevent relapse and recurrence. The mainstay of treatment has been and currently remains pharmacotherapy. However, there is a significant 'efficacy–effectiveness' gap in the reported response rates to all mood stabilizers (Scott, 2001; Scott and Pope, 2002) and even under optimal clinical conditions, prophylaxis protects fewer than 50% of individuals with BP against further episodes (Dickson and Kendell, 1994). Given this scenario, the development of specific psychological therapies for BP appears a necessary and welcome advance. However, until recently, progress in this area was slow.

Historically, individuals with BP were not offered psychological therapies for three main reasons (Scott, 1995). First, aetiologic models highlighting genetic and biological factors in BP have dominated the research agenda and largely dictated that medication was not just the primary, but the only appropriate treatment. Second, there was a misconception that virtually all clients with BP made a full inter-episode recovery and returned to their premorbid level of functioning. Third, psychoanalysts historically expressed greater ambivalence about the suitability for psychotherapy of individuals with BP than those with other severe mental disorders. Fromm-Reichman (1949) suggested that in comparison to individuals with schizophrenia, clients with BP were poor candidates for psychotherapy because they lacked introspection, were too dependent and were likely to discover and then play on the therapist's 'Achilles heel'. Others, particularly clients and their significant others argued strongly in favour of the use of psychological treatments (Goodwin and Jamison, 1990). However, the relative lack of empirical support (prior to the last 5 years, few randomized controlled trials had been published) meant that clinicians had few indicators of when or how to incorporate such approaches into day-to-day practice.

Over the last decade, two key aspects have changed. First, there is increasing acceptance of stress-vulnerability models that highlight the interplay between psychological, social and biological factors in the maintenance or frequency of recurrence of episodes of severe mental disorders. Second, evidence has accumulated from randomized controlled treatment trials regarding the benefits of psychological therapies as an adjunct to medication in treatment-resistant schizophrenia and in severe and chronic depressive disorders (Thase et al., 1997; Sensky et al., 2000). Although there has been only limited research on the use of similar interventions in BP, there are encouraging reports from research groups exploring the role of 'manualized' therapies in this population (American Psychiatric Association, 1994). For persons with BP who reported about a quarter of a century ago that psychotherapy could help them adjust to the disorder and overcome barriers to the acceptance of pharmacotherapy (Jamison et al., 1979), these developments are long overdue.

2. Goals of Cognitive Therapy for bipolar disorders

The main goal of Cognitive Behavioral Therapy (CBT) for bipolar disorder is to maximize adherence with pharmacotherapy and other forms of treatment over time. The empha-sis on attenuation of compliance assumes that even under the best cir-cumstances, most people will be unable to comply perfectly with treat-ment at all times, particularly if treatment is lifelong. If the goals andmethods of treatment are acceptable to patients, the effort of CBT isto increase the likelihood that treatment will be followed as it is pre-scribed. This is accomplished by identification and removal of factorsthat can interfere with compliance.To beneficially affect the course of bipolar, there are at least six separate targets for treatment. The first five of these concern relapse prevention, and the last directly targets the treatment of bipolar depression, see table 1:

1	MEDICATION ADHERENCE
2	EARLY DETECTION AND INTERVENTION
3	STRESS AND LIFESTYLE MANAGEMENT
4	TREATMENT OF COMORBID CONDITIONS
5	TREATMENT OF BIPOLAR DEPRESSION

Table 1. Main targets for CBT to Bipolar Affective Disorders.

The strength of CBT is in altering the course of bipolar disorder over time. Each time a relapse of depression, mania, or mixed states occurs it is an opportunity to learn more about the factors that precipitate recurrences for a given patient. If the patient is not ready to accept the illness, the treatment, and the lifestyle restrictions, CBT will not help.

Sometimes patients have experienced a crisis but have already developed a plan or taken action toward its resolution and merely wish to report to the therapist what has transpired. Telling the story, however, can fill an entire session. When setting the agenda, the therapist should quickly assess whether or not the crisis has been resolved and how much time will be needed for further discussion.

Many institutional settings inadvertently socialize people with bipolar disorder to be passive recipients of care rather than to be active consumers of or participants in their care. A passive view of the patient's role in treatment is in opposition to the collaborative view espoused by this treatment manual. As therapists, we often assume that our patients have basic social skills such as how to get information, how to cope with stress, how to interact with others in various social situations, or how to make decisions about activities of daily living. Some patients who have had bipolar disorder since prior to adulthood may need help to develop these basic skills. These people may have to go through several episodes before they are willing to accept the fact that the illness is recurrent and that they must take control over it rather than letting the illness control them. Involvement of family members in the therapy process can be very useful. It provides family members with an opportunity to meet the therapist and to be informed about what happens during therapy sessions; it demystifies the process of treatment; and it encourages supportive others to be facilitators of care rather than to oppose it. Countering the institutional belief of patients as passive recipients of care can be accomplished by eliciting active participation in the patient. Living through several episodes of depression and mania leaves most people with bipolar disorder feeling fearful and lacking in confidence. The fear is that the symptoms will return especially if they stress or push themselves; see main main objectives of CBT in the treatment of bipolar disorder (Juruena, 2001).

Of individuals with BP, 30–50% also meet criteria for substance misuse or personality disorders, which usually predict poorer response to medication alone. Many of these disorders precede the diagnosis of BP. Bipolar disorder has a median age of onset in the mid-20s, but most individuals report that they experienced symptoms or problems up to 10 years before diagnosis. Thus, the early evolution of BP may impair the process of normal personality development or may lead the person to employ maladaptive behaviours from adolescence onwards. Comorbid anxiety disorders (including panic and PTSD) and other mental health problems are common accompaniments of BP, whilst 40–50% of subjects may have interepisode sub-syndromal depression (Judd et al., 2002). Although many individuals manage to complete tertiary education and establish a career path, they may then experience loss of status or employment after repeated relapses. A period of 1 year after an episode of BP, only 30% of individuals have returned to their previous level of social and vocational functioning. Interpersonal relationships may be damaged or lost as a consequence of behaviours during a manic episode and/or the individual may struggle to overcome guilt or shame related to such acts. The above psychological and social sequelae identify a need for general psychological support for an individual with BP.

However, there is a difference between the general non-specific benefits of combined pharmacotherapy and psychotherapy and the unique indications for psychosocial interventions, see details in table 2. For a specific psychological therapy to be indicated as an adjunct to medication in BP it is necessary to identify a psychobiosocial model of relapse that:

i.   Describes how psychological and social factors may be associated with episode onset. For example, social rhythm disrupting life events may precipitate BP relapse and so stabilizing social rhythms is a key additional element in Interpersonal Therapy as applied in BP.

ii. Provides a clear rationale for which interventions should be used in what particular set of circumstances. For example, the use of Family Focused Therapy (FFT) is supported by research demonstrating that a negative affective style of interaction and high levels of expressed emotion in a family are associated with an increased risk of relapse in an individual with BP.

1	To Educate Patients, Family And Friends About BD, Its Treatment And Difficulties Associated With The Disease
2	To Help The Patient Take A More Participating Role In The Treatment
3	To Teach Methods Of Monitoring Occurrence, Severity And Course Of The Manic-Depressive Symptoms.
4	To Facilitate Compliance With The Treatment
5	To Offer Nonpharmacological Options For Dealing With Problematic Thoughts, Emotions And Behaviors.
6	To Help The Patient Control Mild Symptoms Without The Need To Modify The Medication.
7	To Help The Patient Cope With Stress Factors Which May Either Interfere With The Treatment Or Precipitate Manic or Depressive Episodes.
8	To Encourage The Patient To Accept The Illness
9	To Reduce Associated Trauma And Stigma.
10	To Increase The Protective Effect Of The Family.
11	To Teach Strategies For Dealing With Problems, Symptoms And Difficulties.

Table 2. The main objectives of CBT in the treatment of bipolar disorder.

The need for additional strategies for medication adherence in bipolar disorder is striking. Despite the planned, long-term use of mood stabilizers, a variety of evidence suggests that adherence often fails within the first several months of treatment (Johnson and McFarland, 1996).

The pharmacological management of bipolar disorders faces some of the same challenges of any preventive program of medication; at the time the pill is taken, there may be no disorder-related symptoms, and particularly no symptom relief, to either cue or reward pill taking. Under these conditions, pill use is primarily motivated by the memory of past symptoms and concerns that they may recur. Moreover, emergent side effects may sap this motivation and punish pill taking.

Although all preventive programs may share in these basic factors, bipolar disorder brings additional challenges (Jamison and Akiskal, 1983, Keck et al., 1996). Patients may remember past hypomanic episodes fondly and may desire future episodes. Also, patients may not be convinced of the need for preventive treatment. Under these conditions, it is no surprise that adherence to mood stabilizers is so poor, despite the evidence for a clear link between non-adherence and relapse (e.g., Keck et al., 1998).

A variety of social-psychological research suggests that compliance with requested behaviors is enhanced when an individual's assent to that action is elicited as his or her own opinion (see Cialdini, 1993). That is, it is not the psychiatrist's task to tell the patient why medications are necessary, rather it is her or his task to elicit, with careful questioning, why the patient thinks that ongoing treatment may be helpful. Use of a life-history approach (Post) may be a useful strategy for eliciting relevant patient information on the impact of bipolar episodes on personal and family goals. The life-history method asks patients to construct a timeline of their disorder that depicts manic, hypomanic, and depressive episodes, and the life context that surrounded these episodes. This evidence can then be used to help the patient decide whether an alternative treatment, or greater adherence to current treatments, is a reasonable strategy to adopt.

In focusing on the patient's recommendations in the context of a straightforward and dispassionate presentation of the facts about her or his history of disorder, the prescribing physician will be adopting strategies from "Motivational Interviewing", an empirically supported strategy for enhancing engagement in treatment (Rollnick and Miller, 1995, Yahne and Miller, 1999). Regular adoption of these techniques is encouraged for the treatment of bipolar patients. Moreover, repeated presentation of this information during the initial months of treatment appears to be indicated given evidence for memory and attention deficits in bipolar disorder (Deckersbach et al., 2000b), and evidence that rates of non-adherence are at their average intensity at approximately three months of treatment (Johnson and McFarland, 1996).

Enhancing motivation for medication use is only part of adherence interventions. Indeed a variety of cognitive-behavioral strategies are available to help patients establish a regular habit of medication use. For example, as part of a single-session intervention to improve medication adherence for outpatients with HIV, Safren et al. (2000) recommends the use of imaginal and role-play rehearsal of times and cues for pill storage and use, as well as the use of simple reminders to establish new pill-taking regimens (i.e., colored dots that are placed by the patient in everyday locations – in appointment books, on telephones, in the home bathroom, etc. – that can be a cue for pill taking as well as for reviewing motivation for medication use).

Certainly these strategies can be delivered by independent cognitive-behavioral therapists, but perhaps it is most important for pharmacologists to adopt these strategies directly. At the time of the review of symptoms and diagnosis, the pharmacologist can begin the process of offering expert information on bipolar disorder, combined with a review of the patient's history of disorder and treatment, as part of a motivational intervention. The pharmacologist is engaged in helping establish the patient in the role of a responsible co-therapist on the case, seeking to help the patient define the importance for him- or herself of medication use for control of bipolar disorder. For BD patients, CT always consists of a number of phases. Since BD is a chronic disorder, the educational element is important in facilitating cooperation. The patient is encouraged to ask questions concerning the disorder, its causes and its treatment. As in every type of cognitive therapy, the cognitive model is shown and the patient learns to identify and analyze cognitive changes, as well as automatic thoughts and thought distortions, which occur in depression and mania.

The idea of establishing a cotherapist on the case also extends to other prevention efforts, particularly to efforts at early detection and intervention. In our specialty bipolar clinic, we routinely use a treatment contract and self-monitoring as part of standard pharmacotherapy to formalize the process of engaging the patient in planning for the management of future episodes. The treatment contract itself includes sections that review:

1. The purpose of the contract (aiding the patient in the management of bipolar disorder).
2. Names and contact numbers for other members of the treatment team (including friends or family members who may be asked to intervene at warning signs or crises associated with future episodes).
3. A patient's characteristic symptoms of depressive or hypomanic episodes and the early intervention strategies the patient and her or his treatment team are to enact when faced by these symptoms (Reilly-Harrington et al., 2001).

This contract is an outgrowth of previous work geared towards actively engaging patients in written plans for managing bipolar illness (Bauer and McBride, 1996, Hirshfeld et al., 1997).

Without an organized treatment plan that includes the education and involvement of the patient and significant others, care providers and family members are left to make decisions on behalf of the patient at times of crisis. A treatment contract provides both the patient and clinician with a forum for discussing what the patient would like her or his treatment team to do in the event of early signs of relapse (or a full relapse). The treatment team members should include people with whom the patient has regular contact, and may include health-care providers, family members, significant others, friends, or coworkers. Typically, patients invite family or support system members to sessions focusing on the development of the treatment contract.

After identifying the treatment team, the contract instructs patients to identify specific thoughts, feelings, and behaviors that may serve as early warning signs for episodes of depression and mania. In addition, the patient is asked to outline personal actions to be taken in the event of an impending episode. Of particular importance is the identification of the initial signs of hypomania, to allow early detection and protective action against a potential manic episode. Next, patients develop a set of directives, stating ways in which they and their support systems can be helpful in preventing and managing acute episodes. Strategies of this kind (early detection and intervention) have been found to significantly reduce the rate of occurrence and number of manic episodes (Perry et al., 1999).

Finally, all members of the extended treatment team are asked to review, ask questions, address concerns, and then sign the contract. Once the plan is in place, the clinician(s) and others who apply the contract become agents of the patient's planning, rather than people imposing their own restrictions on the patient.

Even though much of the contract is in a checklist format, it will take time to complete. However, clinicians should consider the contract as an investment against all the time and difficulties associated with future episodes. With the contract in place and relevant contact information and actions pre-specified, clinicians should be able to save time through efficient intervention at times of crisis, or through prevention of future crises.

Current CBT protocols (Basco and Rush, 1996; Newman et al., 2001) also tend to emphasize early-intervention strategies to reduce the impact of hypomanic or manic episodes should they occur. These interventions are designed to reduce the likelihood of poor financial, social, or sexual decisions that may occur in the context of an episode. These strategies range from specification of whom and under what conditions a member of the support network should be able to temporarily cancel a credit card to the specification of rules for risky action. For example, Newman et al. (2001) describe a "Two-Person Feedback Rule", where patients are taught to test out any new plan or idea with at least two trusted advisors. Patients are told of the hypomanic bias of ideas "feeling" good or correct even though they may not "be" correct. With the two-person feedback rule, patients are taught that if an idea really is that good, then two other people should be able to find the idea at least reasonable.

Newman et al. (2001) also discuss a "48 Hours Before Acting Rule" in which patients are encouraged to wait two full days and get two full nights of sleep before acting on any new plan or idea. Patients are encouraged to think to themselves, "If it's a good idea now, it will be a good idea then". This two-day period of reflection also allows an opportunity to put the "Two-Person Feedback Rule" into effect. Any interventions that can potentially disrupt spontaneous or risky decision-making are warranted when working with hypomanic patients.

The approach outlined in Fig. 1 (adapted from Basco & Rush, 1995) is particularly useful when working with individuals with bipolar disorder as it allows the therapist to emphasise a stress-diathesis model that may also include biological factors as precipitants of symptom shift. In order to use this approach, the therapist should first ask about the patient's own views on the causes of the disorder and the associated problems. The patient's aetiological theory is then incorporated within the framework of the model. Links between the individual's cognitions, behaviour, mood and other symptoms (particularly sleep disturbance) and the interaction between these and the environment (stressful events or experiences that are a cause or a consequence of other shifts) are emphasised. This rationale is used to engage the patient in cognitive therapy through monitoring and linking changes in thoughts, behaviours, feelings and the biological symptoms of bipolar disorder. The model also acknowledges that sleep disturbance may be a useful predictor of biological and/or psychosocial disruption and may act as an early-warning sign of shifts from euthymic to abnormal mood states (Wehr et al, 1987). When the connections between the biological and other aspects of their experience are exposed, patients are able to understand the reasons for using cognitive therapy as well as medication. This establishes the rationale for cognitive and behavioural interventions, and also provides a starting point to explore attitudes towards the use of, and adherence to, medication.

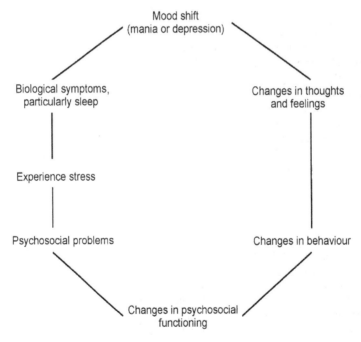

Fig. 1. Conceptualisation of bipolar disorder (adapted from Basco & Rush, 1995).

Keeping an early bedtime schedule is a significant sacrifice for a night person, particularly those who are tired and sluggish in the morning and only begin to find their pace in the late afternoon. If the evening dose of prescribed drugs causes sleepiness, it is often delayed and later forgotten or consciously omitted altogether to avoid the drowsiness that can interfere with activities. Without the protection of mood-stabilizing medications, a recurrence of full-blown mania is almost certain. After years of observation and experimentation, many people with bipolar disorder learn to work with the ups and downs in their mood. They may allow a short flurry of hypomania but know when to put on the breaks, regulate their medication, get some sleep, and slowdown their lifestyle. This is accomplished with varying levels of success. Some wait too long to intervene because they want to enjoy the high or because they do not recognize the mania until they have got-ten into trouble or begin to decompensate. Most hate the lows but feel helpless to stop their progression. More mood-stabilizing medication may not help and can leave them more sluggish. Antidepressants run the risk of inducing mania. Getting medical attention as soon as symptoms of depression begin to emerge is complicated, if not impossible, for most who do not have the advantage of private care and for many who do.

Cognitive processing is also altered during episodes of depression and mania. Speed, clarity, logic, organization, perception, and decision-making ability are compromised. These deficits can have a negative effect on a person's ability to cope with daily hassles and major life difficulties and, in fact, can cause new psychosocial stressors. Improvements in cognitive processing can, therefore, break the evolving cycle of depression and mania at the point of behavior change, impairment in psychosocial functioning, or when psychosocial problems develop.

Although impaired in both depression and mania, the disruption indecision-making ability is qualitatively different in each type of episode. As the cognitive symptoms of depression worsen, self-doubt tends to increase. People do not trust their decisions, fearing failure or disapproval if the "wrong" choice is made. Mental slowing and tunnel vision make it difficult to generate new solutions to problems. And as anxiety increases, it becomes easier to imagine the worst-case scenario for any solutions considered. The magnitude of problems is perceived as great and the consequences overwhelming, and as a result, there is often a paralysis in decision making. Impaired judgment, grandiosity, and impulsivity can all affect the decisions made during hypomanic and manic episodes. Magnification of positives and minimization of negatives can interfere by providing an unbalanced view of the risks and benefits of any plan. It is not unusual for people in a manic phase to act on impulsive urges without pausing to consider alternative actions or solutions. Poor judgment is not always an indicator of impaired decision making. Actions taken in poor judgment can result from a failure to slow down long enough to attempt problem solving.

Activity monitoring and scheduling is a regular component of many cognitive-behavioral treatments of depression (Beck, 1995, Beck et al., 1979, Nezu et al., 1998). Monitoring is used to identify whether the patient suffers from under or overactivity, and whether the patient has a structure for providing breaks and pleasurable events during the week. In depression treatment, efforts are devoted to helping the patient construct a schedule that allows for rewarding activities in areas of both productivity and pleasure, and that helps a patient restart a program of activity if depression has waylaid this area of functioning.

For the management of bipolar disorder, lifestyle management also includes attempts to protect the sleep/wake cycle, to provide a balance in the patient's level of activities, and to monitor for increases in activity that may herald a hypomanic episode.

For sleep management, therapeutic progress proceeds in two stages. In the first, the clinician educates the patient about the role of disruptions in the sleep/wake cycle in heralding new episodes, and discusses with the patient what level of activity and sleep seems most reasonable for the patient. Once the desired hours of sleep have been identified, the clinician should help the patient calculate a regular bed time relative to daily demands and waking times. To aid compliance, the clinician should also identify cues for that target bedtime (e.g., if the patient finds herself watching television to the end of "Letterman", the sleep time has been ignored).

Also, to reduce the impact of other risk factors for episodes—namely, family stress and the impact of negative events—stress management procedures that include training in problem solving, communication skills, and cognitive-restructuring may be valuable. Given that these procedures are a regular part of cognitive-behavioral treatments for depression, these skills may be introduced in the context of interventions for bipolar depressive episodes.

People who have bipolar disorder have daily hassles with which to deal just as everyone else does. They must try to stay on top of problems to keep them from accumulating while they contend with their mental illness and their day-to-day responsibilities. Keeping stress under control may require periodic assessments of life circumstances and regular efforts at solving problems.

Although people make decisions every day without going through each step in the problem- solving sequence, there are times when casual decision making does not adequately address the issues. The most common time to use formal problem solving is when there are obvious difficulties in everyday activities, for example, when there are unresolved problems at home, on the job, or in interpersonal relation-ships. Formal problem solving is most useful when (1) the problem persists despite the patient's efforts, or (2) the patient has been unable to identify a reasonable solution to the problem.

During the first few therapy sessions, patients and their therapists can work together to construct Life Charts. The process of constructing a Life Chart can be very educational for the patient, especially when medication noncompliance has predated recurrences of symptoms. The first step in constructing a Life Chart is to draw a reference line in the middle of the page that represents a euthymic or "normal" state. Many patients report that they have never felt "nor-mal"; therefore, the reference line must represent relative normalcy, that is, relative to the extremes of depression and mania that the per-son has experienced. If an individual has had numerous episodes of illness, the construction of a Life Chart may be difficult. In other cases, the course of bipolar disorder does not begin with an easily defined, distinct episode of depression or mania. There may have been problems at school, at home, or on the job, or there may have been some difficulty in getting along with others. It is usually easiest to start with the most recent episode and work backward in time. It can also be helpful for the patient to try to recall hospitalizations or emergency room visits and use these events as reference points for episodes. Reviewing medical records or talking with family members can also help flesh out the patient's course of illness for a Life Chart.

Another way in which the CBT approach to compliance differs from traditional behavioral contracting is that no external reward is provided. The focus of the intervention is on patients being consistent with treatment because it makes them feel better. Clinicians can help, but taking medications regularly is ultimately the responsibility of the patient. The consequences for noncompliance are internal and personal. The rewards for compliance must be as well. The behavioral contracting intervention for improving compliance begins with a clear definition of treatment plans or goals.

2.1 Treating comorbidity

High rates of psychiatric comorbidity typify patients with bipolar disorder. For example, in a study of 288 outpatients with bipolar disorders, McElroy et al. (2000) found that 42% met criteria for a comorbid anxiety disorder, 42% for comorbid substance use disorder, and 5% for an eating disorder. These disorders were not differentially prevelant among those with bipolar one compared to bipolar II disorder, and in general these findings replicated those from a number of epidemiologic studies (e.g., Chen and Dilsaver, 1995, Kessler et al., 1997).

Treatment of comorbid conditions is an additional role for CBT. For example, anxiety comorbidity in bipolar disorder is associated with longer times to remission (Feske et al., 2000), underscoring the potential importance of managing this comorbidity as part of an overall treatment strategy. At present, CBT and pharmacotherapy (particularly, treatment with antidepressants) represent the treatment modalities with the best empirical support for efficacy with anxiety disorders. Specifically, CBT has been shown to rival or surpass the efficacy of medication in meta-analytic reviews of the anxiety literature, and tends to offer longer-term maintenance of treatment gains (Christensen et al., 1987, Gould et al., 1995,). In many treatment contexts, patients can choose from these empirically-supported alternatives based on preference and availability. However, patients with bipolar disorder may be greatly limited in the choice of pharmacologic strategies for anxiety disorders by the risk of induction of manic episodes associated with antidepressant use. Moreover, there is initial evidence that bipolar patients with significant anxiety may have more difficulties with medication side-effects. As a consequence, CBT has the potential to offer bipolar patients effective treatment without the risk of medication-induced manic episodes or the limitations associated with pharmacotherapy side effects.

Major life events are associated with increased stress and can precipitate an exacerbation of symptoms in the patient with bipolar disorder. Stressful events, especially catastrophic events such as the death of a friend or family member, severe financial crises, major accidents, or ill-nesses in patients or their significant others, can tax a patient's internal coping resources. Positive life events can also be stressful. They require alterations in routine, including eating and sleeping patterns, and may affect symptom control. During these times, the patient may need to rely on more formal problem-solving strategies to cope with the changes associated with the event. Life changes generally have an impact beyond the arena in which they are occurring. For example, job changes can affect life at home and vice versa. Periods of change, therefore, are also times in which more formal problem solving can be useful. Expected role transitions can be similarly stressful and place the patient at increased risk for an exacerbation of symptoms. Role transitions can affect the patient directly (e.g., getting married) or indirectly by means of changes in other family members (e.g., the youngest child moving away from home).

Developmental role transitions, like any other change or event, can be disruptive to the patient's mental health. One reason that life transitions produce stress is that they often change the amount and content of interactions and communication between patients and their significant others. In the next chapter, common interpersonal problems experienced by people with bipolar disorder are covered, including methods for preventing and resolving relationships stresses.

2.1.1 Cognitive model of bipolar disorder

CT's approach to the treatment of bipolar disorder is based on many underlying assumptions. The first assumption is that thoughts, feelings and behaviors of individuals are strongly connected, each influencing the other. Changes in mood and changes in cognitive process, beginning with depression and mania, would inevitably influence behavior. The behavioral responses can reinforce the process of defective information and affective states that have prompted the behavior - a kind of self-fulfilling prophecy.

As noted, CBT has a long history of success in the treatment of unipolar depression. These methods (e.g., Beck, 1995, Beck et al., 1979, Nezu et al., 1998) are also being applied to bipolar depression. For example, in a small pilot study, Zaretsky et al. (1999) found similar reductions in depressed mood for CBT applied to patients with bipolar depression as compared to patients with unipolar depression, see details in table 3. These core strategies are followed by a much broader package of emotional and social problem-solving strategies, combined with modules that target specific difficulties patients may have with emotional regulation, assertiveness, or comorbid anxiety disorders (see also, Henin et al., 2001).

1.	Patients are usually not acute patients during the educational sessions and skills training
2.	Skills will be taught in a didactic manner
3.	Only few cognitive-behavioral techniques will be taught
4.	The agenda for each session is a protocol conducted in opposition to the conduct of the patient

Table 3. CT for bipolar disorder differs from more traditional forms of cognitive therapy.

Early in treatment, patients are provided with a model of the disorder and a rationale for treatment procedures, combined with instruction in a cognitive-behavioral model of the interplay between thoughts, feelings, and behavior. Patients are asked to then complement this didactic information by observing their own experiencing, testing the model, and identifying for themselves the role of thoughts in particular in influencing mood. Each session is presented in a problem-solving format that includes review of the previous week's learning, formulation of an agenda for the session, completion of the agenda with attention to in-session practice of concepts, and then assignment of home practice of skills.

This format maintains a consistent focus on the step-by-step, goal-oriented, skill-acquisition approach that is at the heart of cognitive-behavioral treatments (e.g., Beck, 1995). To make treatment accessible to patients, attention is placed on the use of vivid metaphors and stories to crystallize important information on the nature of the disorder, the process of change, or a specific assignment or skill.

What varies greatly across patients is the quality of their moods, the actions they take in response to symptoms, and the sequence in which their symptoms emerge. Even within individuals the symptoms of mania and depression can change from one episode to the next. Symptoms create impairment. Impairment causes problems. And problems increase stress and exacerbate symptoms. Despite having considerable experience with the illness, not everyone is skilled at identifying the signs of relapse. Early intervention is generally considered the key to control, see figure 2. Waiting until symptoms cluster into a syndrome more likely predicts a difficult course back to normalcy.

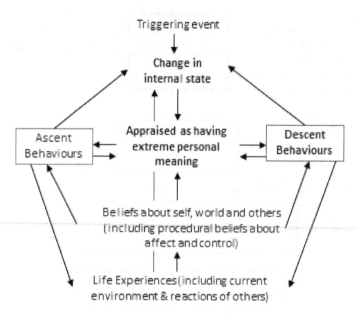

Fig. 2. Cognitive Model of Bipolar Disorder.

The expectation is that by reading this book either therapists will experiment with the psychotherapeutic methods described here in and learn to provide psychotherapy for their patients with bipolar dis-order or clinicians of a variety of types, including psychiatrists, will implement selected interventions with their patients in the limited time available during a medication visit, crisis intervention session, inpatient or day treatment groups, or the course of another type.

What is common among people who suffer from bipolar disorder is its recurrent nature. Once diagnosed, the individual can count on a future of episodic bouts of depression and/or mania that may present in times of stress or change or may recur without provocation. Reasons for hope: Every year there are new developments in the treatment of bipolar disorder. Medications are safer, cause fewer side effects, and provide more positive effects. Psychotherapies have been developed that enhance outcomes, reduce relapse, and aid adaptation to the illness. Given the episodic and recurring nature of bipolar disorder, psycho- therapies, such as CBT, can aid in the anticipation and prevention of future episodes by teaching early detection methods, stress manage-ment, and problem solving.

Early in treatment, patients are provided with a model of the disorder and a rationale for treatment procedures, combined with instruction in a cognitive-behavioral model of the interplay between thoughts, feelings, and behavior. Patients are asked to then complement this didactic information by observing their own experiencing, testing the model, and identifying for themselves the role of thoughts in particular in influencing mood.

Each session is presented in a problem-solving format that includes review of the previous week's learning, formulation of an agenda for the session, completion of the agenda with attention to in-session practice of concepts, and then assignment of home practice of skills. This format maintains a consistent focus on the step-by-step, goal-oriented, skill-acquisition approach that is at the heart of cognitive-behavioral treatments. To make treatment accessible to patients, attention is placed on the use of vivid metaphors and stories to crystallize important information on the nature of the disorder, the process of change, or a specific assignment or skill.

Communication problems occur between at least two individuals, andit is easier for a therapist to help resolve such problems if both partiesare present. This is not always possible or appropriate, however. Insome cases, the second party is a boss, someone who lives a great dis-tance away, or someone the patient is not likely to see again.In normal daily interaction, it is not usually necessary to impose any structure on communication. Structure is useful when communication is ineffective or exacerbates relationship difficulties, however. When preparing to discuss potentially conflictual issues , it is useful to review the basic rules of the communication game as listed in the following:

-   Be calm: It is counterproductive to attempt to discuss difficult issues when angry or stressed in any way. An angry person may let emotions dictate the choice of words and the solutions offered. Solutions that seem reasonable in the heat of anger may prove inappropriate when examined later. It is better to wait until the emotion subsides than to risk making bad decisions.
-   Be organized: It is best to approach the discussion of trouble-some issues after having taken the time to think through what the problem is and what must happen in order to resolve it. Furthermore, it is useful to have a plan for discussing the issue.
-   Be specific: Global complaints (e.g., "I'm not happy," "You're irresponsible,") cannot be easily resolved. It is necessary to specify the action, event, or process that is problematic: What does it look like? How would I know it was happening if I were watching you? What causes the discomfort?
-   Be clear: Beating around the bush or speaking in vague terms leaves much room for misinterpretation of the message. It may appear that the intended message was received, but the message may not have been received accurately.
-   Be a good listener: The best way to be heard is to be a respectful listener. Attentive listening without interrupting is important. The listener should not merely use the other person's talking time as an opportunity to prepare a response (or defense).
-   Be flexible: The resolution of problems between individuals requires give and take. Although a plan to resolve the problems may have been developed before the actual discussion began, it is important to consider others' ideas before selecting a solution. Moreover, others are likely to have a different view of the problem, and all participants should approach the discussion as if the others' perspective is as valid as their own.

- Be creative: In generating a solution to a specific problem, it is useful to look beyond strategies used in the past, to be imaginative, and to try out new plans. If they do not work, another method can be used.
- Keep it simple: Those with communication difficulties should solve one problem at a time. When discussing a problem, they should describe it as simply as possible. If the conversation begins to digress into other areas, stop and redirect the conversation back to the original topic.

The most common source of disruption in communication is emotion.As discussed earlier, intense emotion such as sadness, frustration, oranger can influence the way in which information is conveyed andreceived. If any person's emotional level becomes uncomfortable orappears to interfere with the interaction, the discussion should stopuntil the intensity of the emotion has substantially decreased. It is essential that a plan be made to resume the discussion at a specified time.

The speed and efficiency of cognitive processing can improveearly in the evolution of mania but disintegrate as thoughts increase innumber and speed. Some people with bipolar disorder say they havetheir best ideas when hypomanic. Feeling free from the inhibitingnature of depression, the mind is open to new ideas and possibilities.Creativity during hypomania can result in taking chances at successotherwise inhibited by pessimism and low self-confidence. There isoften an urge or need for stimulation that comes from changes in rou-tine or activity. If judgment becomes impaired, the changes can createnew problems for the individual such as quitting a job before having anew one available. If the quality of cognitions declines, and the personbecomes disorganized or unfocused, changes are initiated but often not completed, see figure 3.

More often, however, the urge for change in the earlyphases of mania or hypomania manifest themselves in more benignforms such as changing hairstyle, clothing, or jewelry, or rearrangingfurniture at home or work. There can be a shift in interests so thatmore time is allocated to planning or research on the Internet or accu-mulating resources for a new project (Juruena 2004).

3. Psychoeducation

People with psychiatric illnesses do not always receive sufficient information about their disorders or their treatment. Symptoms such as impaired concentration, racing thoughts, distractibility, and anxiety may not always be apparent to clinicians but can reduce a per-son's comprehension or retention of information. Likewise, clinicians may not effectively convey information or may not take sufficient time to educate patients. The jargon used in daily interactions among mental health professionals is often confusing to patient. Patients can some-times recall a diagnosis given in the past but may not understand what it means. They will not always ask for clarification because they are embarrassed to acknowledge that they did not understand a word or expression used to describe their illness or treatment. Some-times health care workers fail to provide adequate information because they believe the patient is incapable of understanding, is uninterested, or has already been informed by a previous clinician. Despite good intentions, learning does not occur if information is not clearly sent and received.

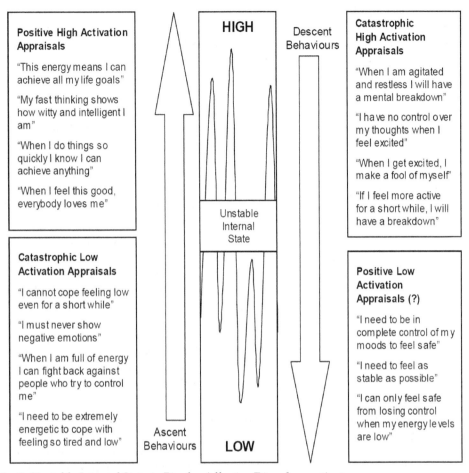

Fig. 3. Unstable Internal State in Bipolar Affective Disorders patients.

The psychoeducational characteristics of CT provide both to patients and to their families and their relationships, learning about what is bipolar disorder, providing and emphasizing the recognition of early symptoms, instructing on the longitudinal course and risk factors relapses and explaining and illustrating the importance and characteristics of treatment and the use of drugs and psychotherapy.

It is noteworthy that both psychoeducation and CBT share in common a focus on medication adherence and compliance,detecting early signs and seeking help. Although these treatments differ significantly in terms of theoretical assumptions, they share some of the same targets and strategies.

Almost all investigations that use CBT involve one or two sessions that provide information about the illness and its treatment,while most psychoeducational approaches include information about lifestyle changes. Both techniques teach patients about prodromal symptoms.

In general, psychoeducative interventions are more informative about illness and treatment,and the content is mainly aimed at improving adherence to treatment. CBT deals more with BD-related residual symptoms of depressive episodes,subthreshold symptoms and negative thoughts,and includes modules on selfesteem, coping skills,assertiveness and life organization.

One limitation of some of the studies examined is the lack of separate comparisons for each block of the intervention (early detection of prodromal symptoms,enhancement of treatment compliance, inducing lifestyle regularity,and so on). With the exception of the study of Perry et al. (1999) that had the advantage of including just one type of intervention,the other studies used several interventions together. In Colom et al. study (2004), psychoeducated patients had higher lithium levels at the 2-year follow-up study compared with control patients,which may suggest an effect of psychoeducation on pharmacotherapy adherence. They used three interventions together,so it cannot be concluded which part was useful,nor can the respective efficacy of each block be determined (Juruena 2001).

Both treatment modes seek to improve the therapeutic approach that is provided in the hospital where research is being conducted, when the control group is _treated as usual. Of course, these traditional treatments are not uniform across the board, although it is generally thought that the only treatment approaches that exist are either supportive or pharmacological. In a detailed study about the impact of an easy-access program, Bauer et al. described how treatment typically consisted of 30-min scheduled medication management visits to a psychiatrist, generally spaced 1–6 months apart. Need for care between appointments was addressed by the psychiatric triage team or the emergency room. Missed appointments were rescheduled at the earliest available time unless a known high-risk situation existed. Other studies do not provide such comprehensive information about how BD is usually treated.

Every contact with patients and their family members is an opportunity to educate them about living with bipolar disorder. The most obvious time is when the initial diagnosis is made. Often this occurs in an emergency room or inpatient unit when the patient is acutely ill. As patients' mental statuses clear, the education process begins. After patients' discharge from the hospital, the education process continues. Because, as was mentioned earlier, the symptoms experienced during the acute phase of treatment may have interfered with patients' abilities to grasp all the provided information, clinicians responsible for outpatient follow-up care can probe for how much information was retained and fill in any gaps. Information will be better retained if everyday experiences are used to illustrate the concepts being taught. Each outpatient visit offers an opportunity for clinicians to inquire about the experiences their clients may have had with the symptoms of bipolar disorder and the treatment. It is common for patients to change health care providers several times during the course of their lives. At each transition point, the education process begins again. Even if individuals previously received care from prominent clinicians with reputations for educating patients and their significant others, those who later care for patients should never assume that further education is unnecessary. Furthermore, as research continues to expand our understanding of the psychobiology and treatment of mood disorders, there will be new information to share (Juruena, 2004).

4. Conclusion

We conclude that preliminary data on CT for BD are promising but more rigorous randomized trials are needed to confirm the efficacy of CT for BD. Another area of research should devote himself to understanding cognitive processes in BD which would allow us to refine and develop unique interventions for this disorder CT, seeking to assess the effectiveness of the cognitive approach, as important as drugs for the TAB.

Overall, it seems that there is promising but not conclusive data about the benefits of psychological treatments in BP. However, there is still much to learn and we need to evaluate whether our current views on psychological therapies in BP fit with the available evidence. For example, the main treatment guidelines on BP, like those on other mood disorders (e.g. American Psychiatric Association, 1993), acknowledge the role and importance of psychological therapies as well as medication. However, the guidelines all suggest that specialist psychological therapies are a precious resource that should therefore be targeted at the most difficult to treat cases. Whilst the notion that those with the most complex problems should be provided with the greatest input seems to make clinical sense, the data from the RCTs reviewed appears to undermine this idea. Persons who appear to consistently benefit from adjunctive psychological therapy are those at high risk of recurrence but do not have other complications or adverse clinical features that commonly accompany BP; i.e. the best candidates for psychological therapies are those with relatively fewer previous episodes, who are at above average risk of a further relapse, but who do not appear to have done well with medication and outpatient support, either because of some ineffectiveness of the prescribed medication or because they are not taking medication. Furthermore, the effect on depression is more marked than the benefit in reducing manic relapses. The latter is of interest because it has implications for psychological models of BP as many of them were initially developed to try to reduce the risk of mania (e.g. FFT to reduce EE and reduce mania; IPSRT to reduce circadian rhythm instability and social rhythm disrupting events and thus reduce manic swings) but appear to have a more overt effect on depression. The theoretical models underpinning the research clearly need to evolve further to m aximize the effect on relapse rates. Further research is also needed to establish whether those individuals with more complex presentations of BP require a longer course of therapy e.g. CBT plus maintenance sessions, or whether a different model of psychological therapy needs to be introduced to help deal with the multiple psychological and social problems they confront over and above managing the consequences of BP.

5. Acknowledgment

To Dr. Paulo Knapp, that have stimulated me to study CBT.

To Professor Ricardo Wainer, for the references.

To Professor Irismar de Oliveira that has shown the mind-brain interface.

6. References

American Psychiatric Association (1994) Diagnostic and Statistical Manual of Mental Disorders, 4th edn. American Psychiatric Association, Washington, DC

Alloy LB, Reilly-Harrington NA, Fresco DM, Whitehouse WG, Zechmeister JS. Cognitive styles and life events in subsyndromal unipolar and bipolar disorders: Stability and prospective prediction of depressive and hypomanic mood swings. J. Cogn. Psychother. Int. Quart. 1999;13:21–40.

Basco MR, Rush AJ. Cognitive-Behavioral Therapy For Bipolar Disorder. New York: Guilford Press; 1996.

Bauer M, McBride L. Structured Group Psychotherapy For Bipolar Disorder: The Life Goals Program. New York: Springer; 1996

Beck JS. Cognitive Therapy: Basics and Beyond. New York: Guilford Press; 1995.

Beck AT, Rush AJ, Shaw BF, Emery G. Cognitive Therapy of Depression. New York: Guilford Press; 1979.

Chen YW, Dilsaver SC. Comorbidity of panic disorder in bipolar illness: evidence from the Epidemiologic Catchment Area survey. Am. J. Psychiatry. 1995;152:280–282.

Christensen H, Hadzi-Pavlovic D, Andrews G, Mattick R. Behavior therapy and tricyclic medication in the treatment of obsessive-compulsive disorder: a quantitative review. J. Consult. Clin. Psychol. 1987;55:701–711.

Cialdini RB. Influence: The Psychology of Persuasion. Revised Edition. New York: William Morrow; 1993;.

Colom F, Vieta E, Martinez-Aran A, Reinares M, Goikolea J M, Benabarre A, Torrent C, Comes M, Corbella B, Parramon G, Corominas J (2003) A randomized trial on the efficacy of group psychoeducation in the prophylaxis of recurrences in bipolar patients whose disease is in remission. Archives of General Psychiatry 60: 402–407

Colom F, Vieta E, Sánchez-Moreno J, Martinez-Aran A, Torrent C,Reinares M, Et Al. Psychoeducation in bipolar patients with comorbid personality disorders. Bipolar Disord. 2004;6(4):294-8.

Deckersbach, T., Reilly-Harrington, N.A., Sachs, G., 2000. Mood and memory in bipolar disorder. Poster presented at the 34th Annual Association for the Advancement of Behavior Therapy, New Orleans, LA, November 2000.

Dickson W E, Kendell R E (1986) Does maintenance lithium therapy prevent recurrences of mania under ordinary clinical conditions? Psychol Med 16(3): 521–530

Ellicott A, Hammen C, Gitlin M, Brown G, Jamison K. Life events and the course of bipolar disorder. Am. J. Psychiatry. Feske U, Frank E, Mallinger AG, Houck PR, Fagiolini A, Shear MK, et al. Anxiety as a correlate of response to the acute treatment of bipolar I disorder. Am. J. Psychiatry. 2000;157:956–962.

Frank E, Swartz HA, Mallinger AG, Thase ME, Weaver EV, Kupfer DJ. Adjunctive psychotherapy for bipolar disorder: effects of changing treatment modality. J. Abnorm. Psychol. 1999;108:579–587.

Fromm-Reichmann F (1949) Intensive psychotherapy of manicdepressives: a preliminary report. Confina Neurologica 9: 158–165

Gitlin MJ, Swendsen J, Heller TL, Hammen C. Relapse and impairment in bipolar disorder. Am. J. Psychiatry. 1995;152:1635–1640.

Goodwin F K, Jamison K R (1990) Manic-depressive illness. Oxford University Press, New York, NY

Henin A, Otto MW, Reilly-Harrington NA. Introducing flexibility in manualized treatment: application of recommended strategies to the cognitive-behavioral treatment of bipolar disorder. Cognit. Behav. Practice. 2001;8:317–328.

Hirshfeld, D.R., Gould, R.A., Reilly-Harrington, N.A., Sachs, G.S., 1997. Short-term cognitive behavioral group treatment for bipolar disorder. Poster presented at the 31st Annual Association for the Advancement of Behavior Therapy Meeting, Miami Beach, FL, November 1997.

Jamison KR, Akiskal HS. Medication compliance in patients with bipolar disorders. Psychiatr. Clin. North Am. 1983;6:175–192.

Johnson RE, McFarland BH. Lithium use and discontinuation in a health maintenance organization. Am. J. Psychiatry. 1996;153:993–1000.

Johnson SL, Miller I. Negative life events and time to recovery from episodes of bipolar disorder. J. Abnorm. Psychol. 1997;106:449–457.

Judd L L, Akiskal H S, Schlettler P J, Endicott J, Maser J, Solomon D A, Leon A C, Rice J A, Keller M B (2002) The long-term natural history of the weekly symptomatic status of bipolar 1 disorder. Arch Gen Psychiatry 59: 530–537

Juruena, MF. Terapia Cognitiva: Cognitive-behavioral therapy for the bipolar disorder patients Revista de Psiquiatria Clínica, v. 28 (6), 322-330, 2001

Juruena, MF . Transtorno Bipolar: Terapia Cognitiva. In: *Terapia Cognitivo-comportamental na Prática - Princípios Científicos e Técnicos* Knapp, WP. (Org.), 317-27, Porto Alegre: Artmed, 2004,

Keck PE, McElroy SL, Strakowski SM, Stanton SP, Kizer DL, Balistreri TM, et al. Factors associated with pharmacologic noncompliance in patients with mania. J. Clin. Psychiatry. 1996;57:292–297.

Keck PE, McElroy SL, Strakowski SM, West SA, Sax KW, Hawkins JM, et al. 12-Month outcome of patients with bipolar disorder following hospitalization for a manic or mixed episode. Am. J. Psychiatry. 1998;155:646–652.

Kessler RC, Rubinow DR, Holmes C, Abelson JM, Zhao S. The epidemiology of DSM-III-R bipolar I disorder in a general population survey. Psychol. Med. 1997;27:1079–1089.

Lam DH, Bright J, Jones S, Hayward P, Schuck N, Chisholm D, et al. Cognitive therapy for bipolar disorder—a pilot study of relapse prevention. Cognit. Ther. Res. 2000;24:503–520.

Lam DH, Watkins E R, Hayward P, Bright J, Wright K, Kerr N, Parr-Davis G, Sham P (2003) A randomized controlled study of cognitive therapy for relapse prevention for bipolar affective disorder: outcome of the first year. Archives of General Psychiatry 60: 145–152

McElroy SL, Atshuler LL, Suppes T, Keck PE, Frye MA, Denicoff KD, et al. Axis I psychiatric comorbidity and its relationship to historical illness variables in 288 patients with bipolar disorder. Am. J. Psychiatry. 2000;159:420–426.

Miklowitz D J, George E L, Richards J A, Simoneau T L, Suddath R L (2003) A randomized study of family-focused psychoeducation and pharmacotherapy in the outpatient management of bipolar disorder. Arch Gen Psychiatry 60(9): 904–912

Newman, C.F., Leahy, R.L., Beck, A.T., Reilly-Harrington, N.A., Gyulai, L., 2001. Bipolar disorder: a cognitive therapy approach. American Psychological Association, Washington, DC.

Nezu AM, Nezu CM, Trunzo JJ, McClure KS. Treatment maintenance for unipolar depression: relevant issues, literature review, and recommendations for research and clinical practice. Clin. Psychol. Sci. Practice. 1998;5:496–512.

O'Connell RA, Mayo JA, Flatlow L, Cuthbertson B, O'Brien BE. Outcome of bipolar disorder on long-term treatment with lithium. Br. J. Psychiatry. 1991;159:123–129.

Perry A, Tarrier N, Morriss R, McCarthy E, Limb K. Randomised controlled trial of efficacy of teaching patients with bipolar disorder to identify early warning signs or relapse and obtain treatment. Br. Med. J. 1999;318:149–153.

Reilly-Harrington, N.A., Kogan, J.N., Sachs, G.S., Otto, M.W., 2001. Treatment contracting in cognitive-behavior therapy: application to the management of bipolar disorder. Manuscript under review.

Rollnick S, Miller WR. What is motivational interviewing?. Behav. Cognit. Psychother. 1995;23:325–334.

Safren SA, Otto MW, Worth J. Life-steps: applying cognitive-behavioral therapy to patient adherence to HIV medication treatment. Cognit. Behav. Practice. 2000;6:332–341.

Scott J (1995) Review: psychotherapy for bipolar disorder – an unmet need? British Journal of Psychiatry 167: 581–588

Scott J, Garland A, Moorhead S (2001) A pilot study of cognitive therapy in bipolar disorders. Psychological Medicine 31: 459–467

Scott J, Pope M (2002) Self-reported adherence to mood stabilizers, serum levels and their relationship to future admissions. American Journal of Psychiatry 159: 1927–1929

Sensky T, Turkington D, Kingdon D, Scott J L, Scott J, Siddle R, O'Carroll M, Barnes T R (2000) A randomized controlled trial of cognitivebehavioral therapy for persistent symptoms in schizophrenia resistant to medication. Arch Gen Psychiatry 57(2): 165–172

Thase M E, Greenhouse J B, Frank E, Reynolds C F 3rd, Pilkonis P A, Hurley K, Grochocinski V, Kupfer D J (1997) Treatment of major depression with psychotherapy or psychotherapy-pharmacotherapy combinations. Arch Gen Psychiatry 54(11): 1009–1015

Wehr TA, Sack DA, Rosenthal NA. Sleep reduction as a final common pathway in the genesis of mania. Am. J. Psychiatry. 1987;144:201–204.

Yahne CE, Miller WR. Enhancing motivation for treatment and change. In: McCrady BS, Epstein EE editor. Addictions: A Sourcebook For Professionals. Oxford University Press; 1999;p. 235–249.

Zaretsky AE, Segal ZZV, Gemar M. Cognitive therapy for bipolar depression: a pilot study. Can. J. Psychiatry. 1999;44:491–494.

7

Cognitive-Behavioral Therapy of Obsessive-Compulsive Disorder

Aristides V. Cordioli and Analise Vivan
Federal University of Rio Grande do Sul, Porto Alegre
Brazil

1. Introduction

Obsessive-compulsive disorder (OCD) is characterized by the presence of obsessions and/or compulsions that consume time and significantly interfere with the individual's daily routines, work, family or social life, causing marked distress (American Psychiatric Association, 2002). Until the 1980s, OCD was considered a rare disorder. The ECA (Epidemiological Catchment Area) study estimated its prevalence rate between 1.9% and 3.3% during individuals' lifetime (Karno et al., 1988). Studies involving children and teenagers demonstrated a prevalence of up to 4.0% (Fontenelle et al., 2006), with slightly superior rates in boys at a 3:2 ratio, possibly due to the more premature symptoms in males (Rassmussen & Eisen, 1992; Walitza et a., 2011).

OCD is a chronic neuropsychiatric disorder and the symptoms wax and wane along its course. The possibility of complete remission without treatment is considered to be extremely low (Skoog & Skoog, 1999). The disorder significantly interferes with individuals' quality of life, with some studies pointing to an impairment level similar to schizophrenia, resulting in incapacitation in the most severe cases of the disorder. OCD was ranked as the tenth cause of years lived in disability worldwide in the Global Burden of Diseases study (Murray & Lopez, 1996). Until recently it was considered a very difficult-to-treat disorder. This point of view radically changed over the last three decades with the introduction of new and effective methods of treatment: exposure and response prevention (ERP) therapy or cognitive-behavioral therapy (CBT) and anti-obsessive medications. Notwithstanding this progress, OCD is still underdiagnosed in clinical practice, since several patients do not recognize the disorder's symptoms and health professionals do not investigate them regularly during the patient's clinical evaluation.

The symptoms of OCD are usually heterogeneous and it is unclear if it is a single disorder or a group of disorders with common characteristics (such as, for instance, intrusive thoughts and repetitive behaviors). In practice, clinical manifestations, age at symptom's onset, course, neurophysiological, neuropsychological and cognitive aspects, as well as response to treatment, vary greatly from individual to individual. A wide range of comorbidities are usually associated with OCD, the most frequent being major depressive disorder, and other anxiety disorders such as social phobia and specific phobias and tics (Flament et al., 1988; Fontenelle et al., 2006; Ruscio et al., 2010; Torres et al., 2006; Kessler et al., 2005).

1.1 Subtypes

OCD patients have distinct clinical presentations. Factor analytic studies have consistently identified five subgroups of symptoms: (a) contamination obsessions and washing/cleaning compulsions; (b) obsessions about responsibility for causing harm or making mistakes and checking compulsions; (c) obsessions about order and symmetry and ordering/arranging compulsions; (d) repugnant obsessional thoughts concerning sex, religion and violence along with mental compulsive rituals and other covert neutralizing strategies, and (e) hoarding (Abramowitz et al., 2010; Leckman et al.,1997; Mataix-Cols et al., 2005). Some suggest that hoarding should be considered a distinct disorder from OCD, with its own diagnostic criteria in the next edition of the Diagnostic and Statistical Manual of Mental Disorders (DSM-V) (Pertusa et al., 2010; Leckman et al., 2010).

Most patients, however, present a combination of the different dimensions of symptoms, although a specific subtype may predominate. Moreover, it is also common that, throughout an individual's lifetime, the symptoms alternate. For instance, a patient who presents predominance of checking rituals today may, during his/her childhood, have had mainly washing or ordering behaviors.

1.2 Etiology

There is strong evidence that neurobiological factors (brain and genetic factors) make certain individuals more susceptible to the development of OCD. The increased prevalence of obsessive-compulsive (OC) symptoms in relatives is well documented, especially among identical twins, which suggests the influence of genetic factors in the disorders etiology (Hettema et al., 2001; Nestadt et al., 2010). Furthermore, the reduction of the symptoms with the use of clomipramine or selective serotonin reuptake inhibitors (SSRIs), the hyperactivity of brain circuits involving the frontal cortex, the thalamus and the striatum, the arising of the obsessive-compulsive symptoms during cerebral diseases like encephalitis or after cranioencephalic traumas or even during the use of certain medications, all point to the involvement of the brain in the physiopathogeny of the disorder.

On the other hand, psychological factors such as faulty learning, distorted beliefs, and catastrophic thoughts are present in most patients, and seem to play an important role in the appearance and maintenance of symptoms.

2. Theoretical grounds of the cognitive-behavioral therapy

2.1 A brief history

Until the 1960s, the main model for the treatment of OCD was based upon Freud's psychoanalytic theory. The obsessive neurosis, as it was known then, was described as a manifestation of unconscious conflicts related to the anal stage of psychosexual development. The proposed treatment was psychoanalysis or psychoanalytic therapy which, in practice, was ineffective in eliminating the symptoms. The dissatisfaction with such an approach led many authors with a behavioral background to undertake some experiments which were crucial to the present understanding of OCD and the development of new treatment approaches.

2.2 The behavioral model

Mowrer's two-stage or two-factor model (1939) to explain the origins of fear and the avoidance behaviors in anxiety disorders has been adapted in order for one to understand the origins and maintenance of OC symptoms. According to this model, symptoms are originated by classical conditioning: the anxiety associated with the obsessions would be paired to previously neutral objects, places and situations (ex.: public bathrooms, bus seats, numbers, colors), which would then evoke it through conditioning. In a second stage the rituals and the avoidance would be maintained because they reduce or eliminate the anxiety and discomfort, albeit temporarily, reinforcing such behaviors and perpetuating the disorder (operant conditioning - negative reinforcement), and prevent its natural disappearance due to habituation (Salkovskis et al., 1998).

2.2.1 The habituation phenomenon

English authors, in the early 1970s, decided to challenge Freud's proposed model, as well as its derived corollaries such as, for instance, that the symptoms, if removed, would be inevitably replaced by others, or that patients could develop a psychotic condition if they were prevented from performing their rituals. They attempted to observe, in volunteers, what could occur if they refrained from performing their rituals or were stimulated to make contact with what they were usually avoiding by reason of their fears.

In a first study, Hodgson and Rachman (1972), while observing patients with cleaning obsessions and washing rituals, found out that they demonstrated rapid and accentuated increase of anxiety when they were asked to touch objects they used to avoid. This anxiety also rapidly decreased when they performed a "satisfactory" washing. In a similar experiment with "checkers" patients, Röper et al. (1973) observed in the same way an immediate increase in anxiety followed by an accentuated decrease after the performance of a checking ritual. Based on these findings, they suggested that there is a functional relation between compulsions and obsessions: compulsions are performed to relieve the anxiety associated to obsessions. This was their function and, at the same time, a tactic learned by the patient to get rid of the anxiety which usually accompanies their obsessions. It is believed that the relief obtained in performing compulsions and with avoidance behaviors is the main factor responsible for the perpetuation of OCD symptoms. The studies also pointed out that the impulse of checking or washing disappeared spontaneously within a 15-180 minute period if patients were requested to refrain from performing the rituals or to remain in contact with the avoided situations or objects. Moreover, at each repetition of the exercises, the intensity of the anxiety and the impulse to perform the rituals decreased. In the case that they repeated the exercises enough times, both the anxiety and the need to perform the rituals disappeared completely. This natural phenomenon became known as habituation and became the basis of ERP therapy. Clinical trials undertaken in the 1970s (Marks et al., 1975; Foa & Goldstein, 1978) proved the efficacy of ERP therapy in OC symptom reduction, becoming, from then on, one of the first line of treatments for OCD.

2.2.2 Evidences of efficacy

ERP therapy is efficient in more than 70% of the patients who comply with the treatment. A similar or slightly superior efficacy of ERP therapy in relation to SSRIs was found in several trials and meta-analyses, definitely consolidating it as the first choice of treatment when rituals predominate and the symptoms are light or moderate in intensity (Foa et al., 2005; Abramowitz, 1997; Rosa-Alcázar et al., 2008).

2.2.3 Limitations of the model

Notwithstanding the success attained through ERP therapy in reducing and limiting OC symptoms, some gaps in the behavioral model have become evident. Most patients do not report a relevant history of conditioning which would have originated OC symptoms. The model does not explain why the same individual presents a variety of symptoms of different dimensions and why they modify, waxing and waning over time. It also does not explain why many OCD patients are tormented by aggressive or sexual repugnant thoughts, without having witnessed or committed such acts (Antony et al., 2007).

Despite the promising results ERP also presented limitations: it has little effect over patients who predominantly present pure obsessions not associated to rituals, or obsessive ruminations (doubt, scrupulosity). On the other hand, around 30% of the patients either abandon the treatment or do not accomplish the homework assignments, especially when the symptoms are severe, or when there is limited insight or overvalued ideas into the contents of the obsessions.

The need to overcome the limitations of the behavioral model and the ERP therapy has led cognitive authors to focus their attention on distorted thoughts and dysfunctional beliefs with catastrophic content present in greater or lower intensity in most individuals afflicted with OCD, highlighting the role of cognition in the origins and maintenance of symptoms (Salkovskis, 1985, 1989, 1999; Rachman, 1997; Salkovskis et al., 1998; Frost & Steketee, 1999). The hypothesis that such cognitions might be responsible for the elevated degree of anxiety associated with the symptoms was raised, due mainly to the low adherence to treatment and to patients refusing to perform the ERP homeworks, and that its correction through cognitive techniques might improve the treatment efficacy. The addition of cognitive techniques to ERP, which has actually always been seen as complementary to the behavioral techniques, has proven useful, especially in patients with obsessive ruminations and predominance of obsessions of repugnant content, in which it is common to find distorted evaluation about threat, distorted believes about danger, responsibility, need for certainty or the so-called fusion of thought and action, with little insight but with good introspective capacity. This addition resulted in the creation of CBT which has gradually been adopted in OCD treatment.

2.3 The cognitive-behavioral model

Today, the cognitive-behavioral model is considered to be the psychological model of OCD with the strongest empirical support (Abramowitz et al., 2009). According to Rachman and de Silva (1978), most people, even those who are not afflicted with OCD, have their minds invaded by improper thoughts of aggressive, obscene or sexual nature, very similar in content to those that torment the OCD patients. However, they do not give any importance to such thoughts and do not attribute any special meaning to their presence; for this reason they easily disappear and do not result in a greater affliction. Still according to the authors, the special catastrophic meaning attributed to the presence of such thoughts ("If I have such thoughts, I can perform them" or "If I think about them, it is because I wish to perform them" or "They reveal a secret and perverse side of my character") is responsible for transforming normal intrusive thoughts into obsessions (Rachman & de Silva, 1978; Rachman, 1997). Rachman's theory, although of great help to the comprehension and treatment of patients tormented by thoughts of repugnant content, does not explain why certain individuals attribute special meaning to such thoughts, while others do not.

Salkovskis et al. (1998) presented an enhanced cognitive model in which they consider the excess of responsibility as a central issue to the origin of obsessions. According to the authors, hypersensitive individuals, due to genetic, neurobiological or environmental factors, present a higher predisposition for catastrophic interpretations. The patient's belief that he/she has the responsibility for preventing future harm to him/herself and especially to others is the crucial ingredient that would lead him/her to perform safety behaviors intended to neutralize such potential risks, such as rituals, avoidance behaviors and checking. The obsessions would persist while the erroneous and distorted beliefs persist, and would decrease when such interpretations weakened. Likewise, the lower the importance attributed by the patients to intrusive thoughts, the lower the impulse to perform the rituals. More recently, Barrera and Norton (2011) investigated a sample of 326 students, and their results corroborate the model previously proposed, concluding that the evaluation of intrusive thoughts is an important predictor of OC symptoms.

A complement of this theory was proposed recently by Rachman (2002) in order to explain the origins of compulsions. Based on Salkovskis's proposition that inflated responsibility would be the central issue of OCD, the author formulated an explanatory hypothesis to the origins of compulsions. They would be repetitive, stereotypical and intentional actions performed by the patient with the intention of preventing future disasters. They would, nonetheless, be some sort of preventive behavior and, in general, associated with indecision and doubt. According to Rachman, checking rituals would be performed when a person who believes to have a big or special responsibility in preventing damage, especially in relation to others, feels insecure that the risk of potential damage may have been effectively reduced or removed, which would lead to repetitive checking as the means of eliminating doubt and possible risk.

2.3.1 Dysfunctional beliefs in OCD

Although Salkovskis emphasized the importance of responsibility, several cognitive-behavioral theorists proposed that the following beliefs domains could contribute to the origins and maintenance of OCD symptoms: (1) inflated responsibility, (2) over-importance of thoughts, (3) excessive concern about the importance of controlling one's thoughts, (4) overestimation of threat, (5) intolerance of uncertainty and (6) perfectionism (Obsessive-Compulsive Cognitions Working Group, 1997). Some cognitive authors also suggested and adapted cognitive techniques, originally proposed by A. Beck for the treatment of depression and anxiety disorders to the treatment of OCD symptoms (Salkovskis, 1985, 1999; van Oppen & Arntz, 1994; Freeston et al., 1996; Salkovskis et al., 1998).

Freeston et al. (1996) found several common characteristics between patients who benefited from cognitive interventions: (1) they greatly value the presence of their obsessions; (2) they believe that their obsessions reflect their true nature (character); (3) they believe that a thought, image or impulse is equivalent to putting it into practice; (4) they believe that having a certain thought increases the odds of it actually happening. Nowadays, more and more cognitive techniques have been added to ERP therapy, and the designation of CBT has been gradually adopted.

2.3.2 Evidence of efficacy of cognitive therapy in OCD

The efficacy of the isolated use of cognitive therapy in the treatment of OCD has been observed in several clinical trials and in at least one meta-analysis, both in patients with predominant obsessions, considered to be refractory to ERP therapy, and in patients with obsessions and compulsions. The results were considered similar to ERP therapy (Emmelkamp & Beens, 1991; van Balkom et al., 1994; van Oppen et al., 2005; McLean et al., 2001).

Some of these studies, however, have been criticized: there was less time dedicated to behavioral therapy than to cognitive therapy. There was also the question as to what extent the therapy had indeed been purely cognitive, if this was actually possible, and if the therapists had not, even indirectly, suggested homework assignments, and if it was ethical to request that the patients did not attempt to do expositions or refrain from performing rituals. In practice, the isolated use of cognitive therapy has not been consolidated, giving ground, actually, to CBT.

2.3.3 Limitations of the model

Undoubtedly, the cognitive model has allowed a broader comprehension of the obsessive-compulsive phenomena. It has, however, been criticized. Evidence has been inconclusive as to whether the dysfunctional beliefs of OCD patients were specific and distinct from dysfunctional beliefs of patients with other disorders. Tools such as the Obsessive Beliefs Questionnaire (Obsessive-Compulsive Cognitions Working Group, 2005) can hardly distinguish subjects afflicted with OCD from those afflicted by other anxiety disorders. Furthermore, the cognitive model does not explain the reasons why many people perform rituals not preceded by any kind of cognition (obsession). This is very common in individuals who have compulsions to align objects, to do things in a sequenced way or perform certain repetitive behaviors which strongly suggest tics: snapping fingers, looking around, rapping repeatedly, touching, scraping. Likewise, the presence of beliefs in patients with hoarding is very modest and does not seem to play an important role in the origin and maintenance of hoarding symptoms.

Furthermore, until today it has been unclear that the incorporation of cognitive techniques to ERP therapy increases its efficacy, possibly due to heterogeneous samples included in clinical trials, with patients who have different OCD symptom dimensions. There is, however, the clinical impression that, for certain patients and clinical presentations, the use of cognitive techniques may be of great value, as well as for patients who predominantly present obsessions or improper thoughts of sexual, aggressive and blasphemous content and obsessive ruminations, due to their need for certainty. Cognitive techniques may also be helpful for patients with poor insight, or very strict or overvalued dysfunctional beliefs, and who, for these reasons, do not adhere to homework assignments. In such cases, the use of cognitive techniques preceding ERP therapy can reduce the anxiety and improve adherence to ERP exercises.

3. Cognitive-behavioral therapy

The cognitive-behavioral approach to OCD is a structured, brief and focused process. Its goal is to eliminate symptoms through confrontation (exposure) of avoided situations, response prevention (refraining from performing rituals as well as all other neutralization strategies) and to correct faulty appraisals and dysfunctional erroneous beliefs. CBT uses psycho-education, hierarchical symptom list, prescription of behavioral and cognitive home exercises, record sheets and instruments for symptom monitoring, as well as permanent feedback.

When symptoms are mild or moderate and there are no associated comorbidities, CBT is usually brief, lasting for 13-20 sessions, according to the specialists' recommendation (Koran et al., 2007). At the beginning of the therapy, the sessions are weekly and last for approximately 1 hour. As symptoms decrease, the time between sessions can be longer. ERP exercises have as their main objective to develop habituation to stimuli considered to be anxiogenic, while the use of cognitive strategies aims at the correction of automatic thoughts and dysfunctional beliefs, possibly helping adherence and ERP exercises, as well as cognitive restructuring for patients who have a predominance of obsessions (pure obsessionals, repugnant obsessions, strong and persistent doubting).

CBT begins with the patient's assessment, psycho-education, followed by graduated ERP exercises, cognitive exercises, discharge and relapse prevention. Below we describe each one of the stages.

3.1 Patient assessment

Patient assessment is undertaken through one or more semi-structured interviews, aimed at establishing the main diagnosis and the presence of comorbidities, as well as collecting data regarding symptom history (age at onset, first symptoms, course of disease), symptoms dimensions, interference in the patient's daily life and family, family members with OC symptoms, presence of medical illnesses, previous treatments (and their effectiveness) and use of medication.

It is important to have in mind that obsessions and compulsions may be present in countless other mental disorders (impulse control disorders, eating disorders, drug addictions, pervasive developmental disorder, etc.); a fact which demands attention in regard to the differential diagnosis. Moreover, comorbidity with some disorders such as impulse control disorders, tics or Tourette, or rheumatic fever may point to different subtypes of OCD, which implies a lower response to CBT and demands complementary therapies.

Still during the assessment stage, some clinical features must be investigated that are usually related to the response to treatment. Studies suggest, although not always agreeing, that the response to EPR may be limited or null in patients who present very severe and incapacitating obsessive-compulsive symptoms; severe anxiety or depression; psychosis; active bipolar disorder; schizotypal personality disorder; histrionic or borderline personality disorder; drugs or alcohol addiction; almost delirious or overvalued beliefs about obsessive ideas; poor insight; lack of motivation towards treatment and non-adherence to home ERP exercises (Neziroglu et al., 1999; Hollander et al., 2002; Raffin et al., 2009).

3.2 Starting the therapy

3.2.1 Psychoeducation

Following the confirmation of the diagnosis of OCD, the first step is psychoeducation about OCD, behavioral and cognitive models of OC symptoms and how CBT works. The therapist provides the patient with relevant information, such as types of symptoms (including the definition of obsessions, compulsions, avoidance, neutralization), the etiology of OCD: neurobiological and psychological factors (learning, appraisal and dysfunctional beliefs), course and prognosis, treatment alternatives, etc. It is essential that the patient understand how compulsions, avoidance and other neutralization strategies contribute toward maintaining the disorder to the extent that the reduction of anxiety is a strong reinforcer for these behaviors. They prevent exposure and consequently the natural extinction of anxiety through habituation and disconfirmation of erroneous and catastrophic beliefs.

Psychoeducation can also be applied to the patient's family, when he/she allows it, providing information on the disorder and how they could contribute to the therapy. In a study conducted by van Noppen et al. (1997), patients whose families received some intervention demonstrated superior gains towards those with whom this did not occur, suggesting that family participation in the treatment may be especially useful.

Direct participation of relatives in the rituals, as well as alterations in family daily routine as a result of OCD symptoms, is seen as family accommodation. It is very common for relatives not to know how to behave in the presence of the symptoms displayed by the patient, supporting their rituals, involuntarily reinforcing such behaviors and so interfering in the progress of the treatment. They frequently modify their routines because of the patient's symptoms and demands. The most common behaviors are offering reassurance, answering questions and doubts, waiting for the patient to finish his/her rituals (dressing, bathing) and taking on the responsibilities (Calvocoressi et al., 1995; Storch et al., 2007; Stewart et al., 2008).

3.2.2 Motivation

One of the great problems of CBT is non-adherence to ERP exercises due to the increased anxiety, even if transitory, that they provoke. Thus, an important factor to be dealt with is the patient's motivation. It is necessary to assess to what extent he/she is willing to engage in the therapeutic process and tolerate some increase in anxiety levels inherent to ERP exercises. In this stage, the establishment of a healthy therapeutic bond may contribute to the adherence to treatment.

Studies have demonstrated that identifying the stage of change in which the patient is, and if necessary, using motivational interview in the first sessions, has increased the rates of response to CBT, consequently reducing treatment dropout (Rubak et al., 2005; Meyer et al., 2010). Doubts and ambivalence are natural, but it is essential to resolve them before therapy begins. The motivational interview is a method centered on the client and aims at reinforcing motivating change, encouraging patients to identify and solve their ambivalences in relation to the treatment (Miller & Rose, 2009). Often, in OCD, the lack of motivation and the difficulty in believing in the possibility of changing behavioral patterns (lack of auto-efficacy beliefs) are associated with previous unsuccessful treatments and with overtly intense and crystallized beliefs about obsessions.

3.2.3 Elaboration of a hierarchical symptoms list

If the patient has accepted to undergo CBT, the first task in the therapy is to elaborate a detailed symptoms list, highlighting compulsions and avoidance behavior, which will be very helpful in planning the ERP home exercises. The Y-BOCS Check List may be used to help the elaboration of the symptoms list. The patient is requested to identify, as detailed as possible, the obsessions, compulsions and avoidance perceived throughout the day. It is also important that he/she classify the symptoms by their level of anxiety or discomfort associated with the obsessions or by the level of anxiety or discomfort that he/she supposes to feel when touching objects or facing the situations routinely avoided, or in case he/she refrained from performing rituals when feeling compelled to do so. In order to do that, the patient is requested to attribute a score from 0 to 100 or from 0 to 10, for the level of anxiety provoked when facing the referred situations. A simplified way of doing this is to use a score from 0 to 4, using the following criteria: symptoms with anxiety level of 1 and 2 (mild); symptoms with anxiety level of 3 (moderate) and symptoms with anxiety level of 4 (severe or very severe). This graduation is helpful in choosing the ERP exercises, since it is recommended to start with those that provoke less anxiety, then move on to the more anxiogenic ones. It is essential to propose exercises that the patient feels capable of accomplishing.

3.2.4 Assessment measures

At the beginning of the therapy it is recommended to assess the severity of the symptoms. The scores at baseline serve as reference, and their reduction can be monitored throughout the therapy. The most frequently used scale is the Yale-Brown Obsessive-Compulsive Scale (Y-BOCS) (Goodman et al., 1989), which presents 10 questions; 5 to assess obsessions, and 5 for compulsions, where scores range from 0 (no symptom) to 4 (severe symptoms), with a maximum score of 40 points. The items encompassed are: time, interference, suffering, resistance and the level of control of the symptoms. Another widely known scale is the Obsessive Compulsive Inventory - revised (OCI-R) (Foa et al., 2002), a self-assessment instrument, with 18 questions to evaluate anxiety associated with OC symptoms and severity. It is important that the therapist proceed with the application of the scales in different moments of the therapeutic process, in order to monitor the patient's progress, allowing for occasional adjustments in the therapeutic plan.

3.2.5 Exercises of exposure and response prevention (ERP)

The therapy itself begins with the ERP exercises, which are chosen by mutual agreement between the patient and the therapist, to be done in the intervals between the sessions.

Exposure is the direct or imaginary contact with objects, places or situations avoided due to fear, discomfort or disgust they provoke. It causes an increase in anxiety, which can be very high in the first exposures, but decreases in the course of time. The exercises must be done daily and last for at least 15 to 30 minutes or until the anxiety vanishes completely, which can take up to 3 hours, and must be repeated as many times as possible. The longer the exercises and the more frequently they are performed, the better. Examples of exposure exercises for patients who have contamination obsessions: to touch a doorknob, a handrail or money, a wastepaper basket, to sit on a bus seat, to use a public telephone or bathroom.

Response (or ritual) prevention consists of refraining from performing rituals, or any maneuver intended to reduce or neutralize the anxiety or fear associated with the obsessions. As in exposure, response prevention provokes an initial increase of anxiety, which decreases over time, reducing, therefore, the intensity of the impulse to perform rituals and their frequency. An example of response prevention exercises for patients with contamination obsessions consists in refraining from washing hands after touching money, or from washing their hands when getting home. Other ERP exercises, selected according to the hierarchical symptoms list, consist of refraining from doing any checking, arranging, not attempting to ward off "bad" thoughts, etc. In the case of patients with hoarding, to discard papers, newspapers, magazines, clothes, shoes or other useless or spoiled objects.

The main effect of the exposure as well as of the ritual prevention is the immediate increase of anxiety in the session, which can reach high levels during the first exercises, but decreases until disappearing in an interval usually between 15 to 180 minutes (habituation), and mainly at each repetition of the exercise. The habituation also occurs between sessions. At first, a ritual or an avoidance behavior that the patient has graded as mild intensity (anxiety level of 1 and 2) is chosen from the list of symptoms. In the choice of home exercises it is worth, above all, to consider patient's assessment regarding how much he/she believes to be capable of performing the proposed exercise, making it clear that nothing will be proposed that he/she does not agree with. It is important to make these rules clear because the patients tend to try to get rid of the most severe symptoms, forgetting, many times, to mention the mild ones. Facing mild symptoms at the beginning of the therapy, however, is very important for the therapeutic process. Succeeding in the less anxiogenic exercises helps the patient to feel safe to face the more difficult ones. Furthermore, at the end of the treatment, there may remain residual symptoms, considered to be mild, and the patient may not report or attempt to eliminate them. There is evidence, however, that the persistence of symptoms at the end of the treatment is associated with a higher probability for relapsing (Braga et al., 2010). The objective of the treatment, therefore, must be the complete remission of symptoms, including those that do not interfere much in the individual's daily routines.

Below are some suggestions for the success of ERP exercises:

- Plan the first exercises focusing on compulsions and on avoidance behaviors;
- Start with the easier exercises (symptoms list with anxiety level of 1 and 2) and select those symptoms that the patient believes to have 80% chances of accomplishing (ERP exercises);
- Choose, together with the patient, 6 to 8 ERP home exercises per week;
- The patient must repeat the exercises as many times as possible: the more often, the better;
- Encourage the patient to do the exercises until the anxiety or discomfort decreases completely or for as long as possible;
- Planned exercises are better than unforeseen ones;
- Make patient aware of the neutralization maneuvers (doing mental or hidden rituals - looking fixedly, mental argumentation, praying, counting, repeating dialogues mentally, repeating "the film" or requesting confirmation or reassurance from other people); these maneuvers have the same function as the rituals (reduce or eliminate fears and anxiety) and he/she must refrain from performing them;

- Together with the patient, identify the trigger situations (situations that activate obsessions and compel him/her to perform rituals throughout the day), and aid him/her in developing confrontation strategies, programming the exercises beforehand.

3.2.6 Modeling

In modeling, the therapist uses the learning through observation (social learning), aiming at stimulating the patient to do the ERP exercises. The technique consists of the execution, in front of the patient, of expositions (touching objects) and refraining from performing rituals as a means of motivating him/her to do the same, afterwards inviting him/her to repeat such confrontations. Patients, in general, have an easier time doing the exercises in the presence of other people and, particularly, the therapist. Examples of modeling may include: touching the shoes and then the face, walking barefoot on the office floor, handling objects such as syringes, keys, money, doorknobs, cleaning products, touching the edges of a garbage bin without immediately washing hands.

3.3 Continuing the treatment

3.3.1 Adding cognitive techniques

The cognitive techniques proposed for OCD must, preferably, be introduced in the therapeutic process when the patient is already able to identify the OC symptoms, avoidance behaviors or anxiety-neutralizing strategies, differentiate obsessions and compulsions from normal thoughts and, mainly, when he/she has already begun the ERP exercises, except in situations in which intrusive repugnant thoughts of a repulsive nature (aggressive, sexually improper, blasphemous), scrupulosity or doubts, predominate, or the patient has poor insight, overvalued ideas and low adherence to ERP exercises. In such cases, when appropriate, the therapy starts with cognitive techniques.

In order for the cognitive strategies to have success, it is necessary that the patient have some introspective capacity, be able to think psychologically, and have curiosity in understanding the symptoms more deeply. The patient must be trained in the identification of automatic catastrophic thoughts and dysfunctional beliefs, the activating situations, as well as their emotional, behavioral and physiological consequences. An interesting exercise is the recording of dysfunctional thoughts, their background and consequences. Next, the patient learns how to classify them according to the beliefs domain to which they belong. For instance, a patient who presents avoidance behavior related to touching doorknobs may have beliefs related to overestimating the risks; a checker, to beliefs about responsibility, and so on. After the identification and association of personal beliefs to the respective domains, the therapist will employ different cognitive techniques aiming at modifying distorted or erroneous appraisals and beliefs.

The cognitive techniques employed in the treatment of OCD are, in general, adaptations of those initially described by Beck for the treatment of depression and by Clark for the treatment of anxiety. Among these techniques, besides the identification and recording of automatic thoughts and dysfunctional beliefs, there are the Socratic questioning, the downward arrow, the examination of the advantages and disadvantages (or of the cost-benefit), the pie of responsibility, the examination of the two alternative hypotheses

(Salkovskis et al., 1998), among others. Its most detailed description may be found in manuals of cognitive therapy and in well-known papers (van Oppen & Arntz,1994; Salkovskis et al., 1998), but is not within the scope of the present chapter. These are some suggestions, however, that the therapist may employ freely and creatively in the elaboration of strategies that focus mainly on cognitive restructuring.

3.4 Ending the therapy and relapse prevention

When the majority of the symptoms have been eliminated, spacing sessions may be proposed and, subsequently, ending the therapy can also be considered. OCD is a chronic disorder and it is important to remember that there is the possibility of relapses, mainly in the patients who did not have complete remission of symptoms (Braga et al., 2005). Thus, the therapist will propose ways of preventing them as the early perception of signs that the symptoms may be coming back, and planning some sessions with the therapist, which are called reinforcement sessions. The reinforcement sessions can be planned and occur at the end of the therapy and through periodic follow-up. They are useful for monitoring the maintenance of the therapeutic gains and contribute to the strengthening of the strategies learned in the therapy.

4. Group CBT

Group CBT uses group therapeutic ingredients for influencing treatment results. Several studies have proved the efficacy of group CBT in the treatment of OC as similar to individual ERP therapy or similar to sertraline (Fals-Stewart et al., 1993; Cordioli et al., 2003; Sousa et al., 2006; Jonsson et al., 2009; Jonsson et al, 2011). Follow-up studies have proven that its effects are maintained in the long run, after discharge (Braga et al., 2010; Borges et al., 2011). Group CBT presents a more favorable cost/benefit relation; with costs five times lower than individual therapy, besides making the treatment available to a larger number of people. It is an interesting approach to use in institutions with high treatment demand. Besides, it is supposed that the group focus may improve the adherence to treatment, an important limitation of CBT for OCD.

5. Use of medication

Both psychotherapy and medications present limitations and, occasionally, contraindications. Several studies do not demonstrate additional advantages in the association of medication and therapy. The results of recent studies, however, reinforce the recommendation of the Consensus of Experts for the Treatment of Obsessive-Compulsive Disorder, which suggests the association whenever possible (March et al., 1997). It is interesting, for instance, the observation that CBT seems to be effective even in patients who do not respond or who respond partially to treatments with anti-obsessive medications (Simpson et al., 1999; Tolin et al., 2004; Tenneij et al., 2005).

In some cases, however, one of the two modalities of treatment may be preferred, at least in the beginning of the treatment. The CBT may be the preferred choice for patients who present a predominance of compulsions and avoidance behavior, whose OC symptoms are mild or moderate, who do not tolerate the side effects of the medication or do not accept using them, and who do not present comorbidities which demand the addition of medication. It is also the treatment of choice of pregnant women, or other patients to whom there may be some contraindication in the use of anti-obsessives, as in bipolar disorder. Medications are the treatment of choice when OC symptoms are severe or incapacitating, when severe depressive or anxiety symptoms are present, when there are almost delusional convictions towards the contents of the obsessions, associated comorbidities which demand pharmacological treatment, or the patient refuses or does not adhere to CBT exercises.

6. Conclusion

The behavioral and cognitive models of OCD allow for a better comprehension of the OC symptoms. They also allow for the proposition of a variety of techniques and strategies effective in reducing OC symptoms in most patients and even the possibility of completely eliminating them. These results completely changed the pessimistic perspectives that until recently predominated toward psychotherapeutic treatment of OCD. Much advancement, however, can be made in the development of new strategies that may reach those patients who have not yet benefited from existing treatment. The definition of more homogeneous subgroups, it is believed, may result in more specific treatments, both from a psychotherapeutic and a pharmacological point of view.

Moreover, when it comes to public health, the explanation to the population of the manifestations of the OCD and its early treatment, especially in children and teenagers afflicted with the disorder, as well as a greater availability of the CBT as a public service, are future challenges.

7. References

Abramowitz, J. (1997). Effectiveness of psychological and pharmacological treatments for obsessive-compulsive disorder: A quantitative review of the controlled treatment literature. *Journal of Consulting and Clinical Psychology*, Vol.65, No.1, (February 1997), pp. 44-52, ISSN 0022-006X

Abramowitz, J., Taylor, S., & McKay, D. (2009). Obsessive-compulsive disorder. *Lancet*, Vol.374, No.9688, (August 2009), pp. 491-499, ISSN 0140-6736

Abramowitz, J., Deacon, B., Olatunji, B., Wheaton, M., Berman, N., Losardo, D., Timpano, K., McGrath, P., Riemann, B., Adams, T., Björgvinsson, T., Storch, E., & Hale, L. (2010). Assessment of obsessive-compulsive symptom dimensions: Development and evaluation of the Dimensional Obsessive-Compulsive Scale. *Psychological Assessment*, Vol.22, No.1, (March 2010), pp. 180-198, ISSN 1040-3590

American Psychiatric Association. (2002). *DSM-IV-TR – Manual diagnóstico e estatístico de transtornos mentais* (4ed). Artmed, ISBN 9788573079852 , Porto Alegre, Brazil

Antony, M., Purdon, C., & Summerfeldt, L. (2007). *Psychological treatment of obsessive-compulsive disorder: Fundamentals and Beyond*. American Psychological Association, ISBN 1591474841, Washington D.C., USA

Barrera, T., & Norton, P. (2011). The appraisal of intrusive thoughts in relation to obsessional-compulsive symptoms. *Cognitive Behaviour Therapy*, Vol.1, No.1, (April 2011), ISSN 1651-2316

Borges, C., Meyer, E., Ferrão, Y., Souza, F., & Cordioli, A.V. (2011). Cognitive-behavioral group therapy versus sertraline for obsessive-compulsive disorder: five-year follow-up. *Psychotherapy and Psychosomatics*, Vol.80, (May 2011), pp. 249-250, ISSN 1423-0348

Braga, D., Cordioli, A., Niederauer, K., & Manfro, G. (2005). Cognitive-behavioral group therapy for obsessive-compulsive disorder: a 1-year follow-up. *Acta Psychiatrica Scandinavica*, Vol.112, No.3, (September, 2005), pp.180-186, ISSN 0001-690X

Braga, D., Manfro, G., Niederauer, K., & Cordioli, A. (2010). Full remission and relapse of obsessive-compulsive symptoms after cognitive-behavioral group therapy: a two-year follow-up. *Revista Brasileira de Psiquiatria*, Vol.32, No.2, (June 2010), pp. 164-168, ISSN 1516-4446

Calvocoressi, L., Lewis, B., Hariis, M., Trufan, S., Goodman, W., McDougle, C., & Price, L. (1995). Family accommodation in obsessive-compulsive disorder. *The American Journal of Psychiatry*, Vol.152, No.3, (March 1995), pp.441-443, ISSN 0002-953X

Cordioli, A.V., Heldt, E., Bochi, D., Margis, R., Sousa, M., Tonello, J., Manfro, G., Kapczinski, F. (2003).Cognitive-behavioral group therapy in obsessive-compulsive disorder: a randomized clinical trial. *Psychotherapy and Psychosomatics*, Vol.72, No.4, pp.211-216, ISSN 0033-3190

Emmelkamp, P., & Beens, H. (1991). Cognitive therapy with obsessive-compulsive disorder: a comparative evaluation. *Behaviour Research and Therapy*, Vol.29, No.3, pp.293-300, ISSN 0005-7967

Fals-Stewart, W., Marks, A., & Schafer, J. (1993). A comparison of behavioral group therapy and individual behavior therapy in treating obsessive-compulsive disorder. *Journal of Nervous and Mental Disease*, Vol.181, No.3, (March 1993), pp. 189-193, ISSN 0022-3018

Flament, M., Whitaker, A., Rapoport, J., Davies, M., Berg, C., Kalikow, K., Sceery, W., & Shaffer, D. (1988) Obsessive compulsive disorder in adolescence: An epidemiological study. *Journal of the American Academy of Child & Adolescence Psychiatry*, Vol.27, No.6, (November 1988), pp. 764–771, ISSN 0890-8567

Foa, E., & Goldstein, A. (1978). Continuos exposure and complete response prevention in the treatment of obsessive-compulsive neurosis. *Behavioral Therapy*, Vol.9, No.5, (November 1978), pp. 821-829

Foa, E., Huppert, J., Leiberg, S., Langner, R, Kichic, R., Hajcak, G., & Salkovskis, P. (2002). The Obsessive Compulsive Inventory: Development and validation of a short version. *The Psychological Assessment*, Vol.14, No.4, (December 2002), pp. 485-495, ISSN 1040-3590

Foa, E., Liebowitz, M., Kozak, M., Davies, S., Campeas, R., Franklin, M., Huppert, J., Kjernisted, K., Rowan, V., Schmidt, A., Simpson, H., & Tu, X. (2005). Randomized, placebo-controlled trial of exposure and ritual prevention, clomipramine, and their combination in the treatment of obsessive-compulsive disorder. *The American Journal of Psychiatry*, Vol.162, No.1, (January 2005), pp. 151-161, ISNN 0002-953X

Fontenelle, L., Mendlowicz, M., & Versiani, M. (2006). The descriptive epidemiology of obsessive-compulsive disorder. *Progress in Neuropsychopharmacology and Biological Psychiatry*, Vol.30, No.3, (May 2006), pp. 327-337, ISSN 0278-5846

Freeston, M., Rhéaume, J., & Ladouceur, R. (1996). Correcting faulty appraisal of obsessional thoughts. *Behavior Research and Therapy*, Vol.34, No.5-6, (May-June 1996), pp. 433-446, ISSN 0005-7967

Frost, R., & Steketee, G. (1999) Issues in the treatment of compulsive hoarding. *Cognitive and Behavioral Practice*, Vol.6, No. 4, pp. 397-407

Goodman, W., Price, L., Rasmussen, S. (1989). The Yale-Brown obsessive-compulsive scale (YBOCS) part I: development, use, and reliability. *Archives of General Psychiatry*, Vol.46, No.11, (November 1989), pp. 1006-1011, ISSN 0003-990X

Hettema, J., Neale, M., & Kendler, K. (2001). A review and meta-analysis of the genetic epidemiology of anxiety disorders. *The American Journal of Psychiatry*, Vol.158, No.10, (October 10), pp. 1568-78, ISSN 0002-953X

Hodgson, R., & Rachman, S. (1972). The effects of contamination and washing in obsessional patients. *Behaviour Research and Therapy*, Vol.10, No.02, (May 1972), pp. 111-117, ISSN 0005-7967

Hollander, E., Bienstock, C., Koran, L., Pallanti, S., Marazziti, D., Rasmussen, S., Ravizza, L., Benkelfat, C., Saxena, S., Greenberg, B., Sasson, Y., & Zohar, J. (2002). Refractory obsessive-compulsive disorder: state of the art treatment. *Journal of Clinical Psychiatry*, Vol.63, pp. 20-29, ISSN 0160-6689

Jonsson, H., & Hougaard, E. (2009). Group cognitive behavioural therapy for obsessive-compulsive disorder: a systematic review and meta-analysis. *Acta Psychiatrica Scandinavica*, Vol.119, No.2, (February 2009), pp. 98-106, ISSN 1600-0447

Jonsson, H., Hougaard, E., & Bennedsen, B. (2011). Randomized comparative study of group versus individual cognitive behavioural therapy for obsessive compulsive disorder. *Acta Psychiatrica Scandinavica*, Vol.123, No.5, (May 2011), pp. 387-397, ISSN 1600-0447

Karno, M., Golding, J., Sorenson, S., & Burnam, M. (1988). The epidemiology of obsessive-compulsive disorder in five US communities. *Archives of General Psychiatry*, Vol.45, No. 2, (December 1988), pp. 1094-1099, ISSN 0003-990X

Kessler, R., Berglund, P., Demler, O., Jin, R., & Walters, E. (2005). Lifetime prevalence and age-of-onset distributions of DSM-IV disorders in the National Comorbidity Survey Replication. *Archives of General Psychiatry*, Vol.62,No.6, (June 2005), pp. 593–602, ISSN 0003-990X

Koran, L., Hanna, G., Hollander, E., & Nestadt, G. (2007). Practice guideline for the treatment of patients with obsessive-compulsive disorder. *The American Journal of Psychiatry*, Vol.164, No.7, (July 2007), pp. 5–53, ISSN 0002-953X

Leckman, J., Grice, D., & Boardman, J., Zhang, H., Vitale, A., Bondi, C., Alsobrook. J., Peterson, B., Cohen, D., Rasmussen, S., Goodman, C., McDougle, C., & Pauls, D. (1997). Symptoms of obsessive-compulsive disorder. *The American Journal of Psychiatry*, Vol.154, No.7, (July 1997), pp. 911-917, ISSN 0002-953X

Leckman, J., Denys, D., Simpson, B., Mataix-Cols, D., Hollander, E., Saxena, S., Miguel, E., Rauch, S., Goodman, W., Phillips, K., & Stein, D. (2010). Obsessive–compulsive disorder: a review of the diagnostic criteria and possible subtypes and dimensional specifiers for DSM-V. *Depression and Anxiety*, Vol.27, No.6, (June 2010), pp. 507-527, ISSN 1520-6394

March, J., Frances, A., Kahn, D., & Carpenter, D. (1997). The expert consensus guideline series: treatment of obsessive-compulsive disorder. *Journal of Clinical Psychiatry*, Vol.58, No.4, pp. 1-72, ISSN 0160-6689

Marks, I., Hodgson, R., & Rachman, S. (1975). Treatment of chronic obsessive-compulsive neurosis by in-vivo exposure – a two year follow-up and issues in treatment. *The British Journal of Psychiatry*, Vol.127, (October 1975), pp. 349-364, ISSN 0007-1250

Mataix-Cols, D., Rosário-Campos, M., Leckman, J. (2005). A multidimensional model of obsessive-compulsive disorder. *The American Journal of Psychiatry*, Vol.162, No.2, (February 2005), pp. 228-238, ISSN 0002-953X

McLean, P., Whittal, M., Thordarson, D., Taylor, S., Söchting, I., Koch, W., Paterson, R., & Anderson, K. (2001). Cognitive versus behavior therapy in the group treatment of obsessive-compulsive disorder. *Journal of Consulting and Clinical Psychology*, Vol.69, No.2, (April 2001), pp. 205-214, ISSN 0022-006X

Meyer, E., Souza, F., Hekdt, E., Knapp, P., Cordioli, A., Shavitt, R., & Leukefeld, C. (2010). A randomized clinical trial to examine enhancing cognitive-behavioral group therapy for obsessive-compulsive disorder with motivational interviewing and thought mapping. *Behavioural and Cognitive Psychotherapy*, Vol.38, No.3., (May 2010), pp. 319-336, ISSN 1469-1833

Miller, W., & Rose, G. (2009). Toward a theory of motivational interviewing. *The American Psychologist*, Vol.64, No.6, (September 2009), pp. 527-537, ISSN 1935-990X

Mowrer, O. (1939). A stimulus-response analysis of anxiety and its role as a reinforcing agent. *Psychological Review*, Vol.46, pp. 553-565

Murray, C., & Lopez, A. (1996). *The global burden of disease*. Harvard University Press, ISBN 9780674354487, Cambridge, USA

Nestadt, G., Grados, M., & Samuels, J. (2010). Genetics of obsessive-compulsive disorder. *Psychiatric Clinics of North America*, Vol.33, No.1, (March 2010), pp.141-158 ISSN 1558-3147

Neziroglu, F., Stevens, K., Yaryura-Tobias, J. (1999). Overvalued ideas and their impacto n treatment outcome. *Revista Brasileira de Psiquiatria*, Vol.21, No.4, (December 1999), pp. 209-216, ISSN 1516-4446

Obsessive-Compulsive Cognitions Working Group. (1997). Cognitive assessment of obsessive-compulsive disorder. *Behaviour Research and Therapy*, Vol.35, No.7, (July 1997), pp. 667-681, ISSN 0005-7967

Obsessive-Compulsive Cognitions Working Group. (2005). Psychometric validation of the Obsessive Belief Questionnaire and the interpretation of intrusions inventory: part 2. Factor analyses and testing of a brief version. *Behaviour Research and Therapy*, Vol.43, No.11, (November 2005), pp. 1527–1542, ISSN 0005-7967

Pertusa, A., Frost, R., Fullana, M., Samuels, J., Steketee, G., Tolin, D., Saxena, S., Leckman, J., & Matix-Cols, D. (2010). Refining the diagnostic boundaries of compulsive hoarding: a critical review. *Clinical Psychology Review*, Vol.30, No.4, (June 2010), pp. 371-386, ISSN 1873-7811

Rachman, D., & de Silva, P. (1978). Abnormal and normal obsession. *Behaviour Research and Therapy*, Vol.16, No.4, pp. 233-248, ISSN 0005-7967

Rachman, S. (1997). A cognitive theory of obsessions. *Behaviour Research and Therapy*, Vol.35, No.9, (September 1997), pp. 793-780, ISSN 0005-7967

Rachman, S. (2002). A cognitive theory of compulsive checking. *Behaviour Research and Therapy*, Vol.40, No.6, (June 2002), pp. 625-639, ISSN 0005-7967

Raffin, A., Fachel, J., Ferrão, Y., de Souza, F., & Cordioli, A. (2009). Predictors of response to group cognitive-behavioral therapy in the treatment of obsessive-compulsive disorder. *European Psychiatry*, Vol.24, No.5, (June 2009), pp. 297-306, ISSN 0924-9338

Rassmussen, A., & Eisen, J. (1992). The epidemiological and clinical features of obsessive-compulsive disorder. *Psychiatric Clinics of North America*, Vol.15, No.4, (December 1992), pp. 743-758, ISSN 0193-953X

Röper, G., Rachman, S., & Hodgson, R. (1973). An experiment on obsessional checking. *Behaviour Research and Therapy*, Vol.11, No.3, (Augusti 1973), pp. 271–277, ISSN 0005-7967

Rosa-Alcázar, A., Sanchez-Meca, J., Gomez-Conesa, A., & Marin-Martinez, F. (2008). Psychological treatment of obsessive-compulsive disorder: a meta-analysis. *Clinical Psychology Review*, Vol.28, No.8, (December 2008), pp. 1310-1325, ISSN 1873-7811

Rubak, S., Sandbaek, A., Lauritzen, T., & Christensen, B. (2005). Motivational interviewing: a systematic review and meta-analysis. *British Journal of General Practice*, Vol.55, No. 513, (April 2005), pp. 305–312, ISSN 0960-1643

Ruscio, A., Stein, D., Chiu, W., & Kessler, R. (2010). The epidemiology of obsessive-compulsive disorder in the National Comorbidity Survey Replication. *Molecular Psychiatry*, Vol.15, No.1, (January 2010), pp. 53-63, ISSN 1476-5578

Salkovskis, P. (1985). Obsessional-compulsive problems: a cognitive-behavioral analysis. *Behavior Research and Therapy*, Vol.23, No.5, pp. 571-583, ISSN 0005-7967

Salkovskis, P. (1989). Cognitive-behavioural factors and the persistence of intrusive thoughts in obsessional problems. *Behavior Research and Therapy*, Vol.27, No.6, pp.677-682, ISSN 0005-7967

Salkovskis, P., Forrester, E., & Richards, C. (1998). Cognitive-behavioural approach to understanding obsessional thinking. *The British Journal of Psychiatry*, Vol.173, No.35, pp. 53-63, ISSN 0960-5371

Salkovskis, P. (1999). Understanding and treating obsessive-compulsive disorder. *Behavior Research and Therapy*, Vol.37, No.1, (July 1999), pp. 29-52, ISSN 0005-7967

Simpson, H., Gorfinkle, K., Liebowitz, M. (1999). Cognitive-behavioral therapy as an adjunct to serotonin reuptake inhibitors in obsessive-compulsive disorder: an open trial. *Journal of Clinical Psychiatry*, Vol.60, No.9, (September 1999), pp. 584-590, ISSN 0160-6689

Skoog, G., & Skoog, I. (1999). A 40-year follow-up of patients with obsessive-compulsive disorder. *Archives of General Psychiatry*, Vol.56. No.2, (February 1999), pp. 121-127, ISSN 0003-990X

Sousa, M., Isolan, L., Oliveira, R., Manfro, G., & Cordioli, A. (2006). A randomized clinical trial of cognitive-behavioral group therapy and sertraline in the treatment of obsessive-compulsive disorder. *Journal of Clinical Psychiatry*, Vol.67, No.7, (July 2006), pp. 1133-1139, ISSN 0160-6689

Stewart, S., Beresin, C., Haddad, S., Egan Stack, D., Fama, J., Jenike, M. (2008) Predictors of family accommodation in obsessive-compulsive disorder. *Annals of Clinical Psychiatry*, Vol.20, No.2, (April-June 2008), pp. 65-70, ISSN 1547-3325

Storch, E., Geffken, G., Merlo, L., Jacob, M., Murphy, T., Goodman, W., Larson, M., Fernandez, M., & Grabill, K. (2007). Family accommodation in pediatric obsessive-compulsive disorder. *Journal of Clinical Child and Adolescent Psychology*, Vol.36, No.2, (April-June 2007), pp. 207-216, ISSN 1537-4416

Tenneij, N., van Megen, H, Denys, D., Westenberg, H. (2005). Behavior therapy augments response of patients with obsessive-compulsive disorder responding to drug treatment. *Journal of Clinical Psychiatry*, Vol.66, No.9, (September 2005), pp. 1169-1175, ISSN 0160-6689

Tolin, D. Maltby, N., Diefenbach, G., Hannan, S., Worhunsky, P. (2004). Cognitive-behavioral therapy for medication nonresponders with obsessive-compulsive disorder: a wait-list-controlles open trial. *Journal of Clinical Psychiatry*, Vol.65, No.7, (July 2004), pp. 922-931, ISSN 0160-6689

van Balkom A., van Oppen, P., Vermeulen, A., van Dyck, R., Nauta, M., & Vorst, H. (1994). A meta-analysis on the treatment of obsessive-compulsive disorder: a comparasion of antidepressants, behavior, and cognitive therapy. *Clinical Psychology Review*, Vol.14, No.5, pp. 359-3981

van Noppen B., Steketee, G., McCorkle, B. & Pato, M. (1997). Group and multifamily behavioral treatment for obsessive compulsive disorder: a pilot study. *Journal of Anxiety Disorders*, Vol.11, No.4, (July-August 1997), pp. 431-446, ISSN 0887-6185

van Oppen, P., & Arntz, A. (1994). Cognitive therapy for obsessive-compulsive disorder. *Behavior Research and Therapy*, Vol.32, No.1, (January 1994), pp. 79-87, ISSN 0005-7967

van Oppen, P., van Balkom, A., de Haan, E., & van Dyck, R. (2005). Cognitive therapy and exposure in vivo alone and in combination with fluvoxamine in obsessive-compulsive disorder: a 5-year follow-up. *Journal of Clinical Psychiatry*, Vol.66, No.11, (November 2005), pp. 1415-1422, ISSN 0160-6689

Walitza, S., Melfsen, S., Jans, T., Zellmann, H., Wewetzer, C., & Warke, A. (2011). Obsessive-compulsive disorder in children and adolescents. *Deutsches Aerzteblatt International*, Vol.108, No.11, (March 2011), pp. 173-179, ISSN 1866-0452

8

Cognitive-Behavior Therapy for Substance Abuse

Bernard P. Rangé[1] and Ana Carolina Robbe Mathias[2]
[1]Graduate Program in Psychology, Psychology Institute,
Federal University at Rio de Janeiro,
[2]Psychiatric Institute, Federal University at Rio de Janeiro,
Brazil

1. Introduction

Drug use and drug abuse are old topics that are increasingly current. New drugs and new ways of using them appear all the time, and researchers dedicate more and more time to understanding their mechanisms and effects. The 2008 National Survey on Drug Abuse and Health Survey estimated that 8% of the American population over 12 years of age made use of an illegal drug in the previous year, and that half of this population (56%) stated they currently consumed alcohol (Substance Abuse and Mental Health Services Administration, 2009). The most commonly used illegal drug was found to be marijuana, with 15% of users stating they consumed it daily or almost daily.

When treating a drug user, it is necessary to go beyond the effect that the drug produces on the individual in order to understand how the person deals with the drug, to identify what leads them to use drugs and what role drugs have in their life. With this in mind, Cognitive-Behavioral Therapy (CBT) encourages the individual to become aware of their drug problem, to understand how it affects their daily functioning, and to establish a healthier way of life.

2. Diagnostic criteria

When evaluating a person's substance use problem, two diagnoses should be taken into account: substance abuse and substance dependence. A diagnosis of substance abuse is made when the substance is used in large amounts, and when social, occupational, physical, and family impairments occur which do not keep the individual from continuing to use the substance. On the other hand, a substance dependence diagnosis is made when there is tolerance, withdrawal, loss of control of the amount taken and the time spent, and interruption of important activities (DSM-IV-TR, 2002). This difference is important in deciding how to conduct treatment.

According to the Diagnostic and Statistical Manual of Mental Disorders (DSM-IV-TR, APA, 2002), the diagnostic criteria for substance abuse and substance dependence are as follows:

DSM-IV Substance Abuse Criteria

a. A maladaptive pattern of substance use leading to clinically significant impairment or distress as manifested by one (or more) of the following, occurring within a 12-month period:
    1. Recurrent substance use resulting in a failure to fulfill major role obligations at work, school, or home.
    2. Recurrent substance use in situations in which it is physically hazardous
    3. Recurrent substance-related legal problems
    4. Continued substance use despite persistent or recurrent social or interpersonal problems.
b. The symptoms have never met the criteria for Substance Dependence.

DSM-IV Substance Dependence Criteria

A maladaptive pattern of substance use leading to clinically significant impairment or distress, as manifested by three (or more) of the following, occurring any time in the same 12-month period:

1. Tolerance, as defined by either of the following: (a) A need for markedly increased amounts of the substance to achieve intoxication or the desired effect or (b) Markedly diminished effect with continued use of the same amount of the substance.
2. Withdrawal, as manifested by either of the following: (a) The characteristic withdrawal syndrome for the substance or (b) The same (or closely related) substance is taken to relieve or avoid withdrawal symptoms.
3. The substance is often taken in larger amounts or over a longer period than intended.
4. There is a persistent desire or unsuccessful efforts to cut down or control substance use.
5. A great deal of time is spent in activities necessary to obtain the substance (e.g., seeing different doctors, driving long distances), use the substance (e.g. smoking in the company of others), or recover from its effects.
6. Important social, occupational, or recreational activities are given up or reduced because of substance use.
7. The substance use is continued despite knowledge of having a persistent physical or psychological problem that is likely to have been caused or exacerbated by the substance (for example, current cocaine use despite recognition of cocaine-induced depression or continued drinking despite recognition that an ulcer was made worse by alcohol consumption).

3. Comorbidity

Substance abuse and dependence disorders are often related to other psychiatric disorders. When making a first assessment, it is important to try to identify whether comorbidity is unrelated to substance use or a consequence of it. This can change the course of treatment. For instance, in the case of a patient who abuses alcohol and suffers from depression, their drinking may be a consequence of depression, and thus the treatment should focus primarily on depression; on the other hand, if depression occurred during or after the development of the substance abuse disorder, the former may be a consequence of the latter, and so the treatment should focus more on the abuse problem. However, it is often the case that this assessment can only be made after the substance use ceases, and one can then observe whether the symptoms persist in the absence of the substance.

The main disorders associated to substance abuse and dependence are mood disorders (Swendsen, 2010 et al.; Ilgen et al., 2008) and anxiety disorders, such as social phobia and generalized anxiety disorder (Robinson et al., 2011, Swendsen et al., 2010; Boton et al., 2006). Studies show that other disorders can occur concomitantly with substance use, such as post-traumatic stress disorder (Petrakis et al., 2011), pathological gambling (Mathias et al., 2009) and nicotine dependence (Ferron et al., 2011). In addition to these disorders, the relationship between substance use and suicide is cause for concern (Vijayakumar et al., 2011). This aspect must always be the object of an in-depth evaluation, as it puts the patient's life at immediate risk.

4. Treatment

Cognitive-behavioral treatment of substance abuse must take into account three theoretical principles: Motivational Interviewing (MI), which establishes motivation and commitment to treatment; Cognitive Therapy (CT) for substance abuse, which makes it possible to identify and change thoughts and beliefs that lead the patient to seek drugs and alcohol, and Relapse Prevention (RP), which deals with high-risk situations, leading to better results.

Treatment is successful when the therapist is able to interconnect these three theoretical principles, adjusting them according to each patient's needs.

4.1 Motivational interviewing

MI is an approach developed in the 1980s by William Miller and Stephen Rollnick (2001) specifically to treat patients who were resistant to behavior changes. It is defined as a collaborative and evocative technique that respects the patient's autonomy (Rollnick, Miller and Butler, 2008). Motivation is seen as a changeable phenomenon that can be influenced, constructed and developed within the patient-therapist relationship.

The main point of MI is to work on ambivalence, the feeling of doubt that gives rise to a conflict between wanting/doing and not wanting/not doing something. For a better understanding of ambivalence, the authors made use of the stages of change as developed by Prochaska, DiClemente and Norcross (1992), according to which the patient goes through certain stages in order to achieve the change that is needed.

First, in what is called the pre-contemplation stage, the person does not consider change, or denies the need for it. When the person admits the need for change but is still uncertain as to whether they want to make the change or not, they have moved to the contemplation stage. In this stage, ambivalence is at its peak. After contemplation, the person starts to take some steps in order to change, which characterizes the preparation stage. Then comes the action stage, the moment in which change is put into effect. When change has been established and the person is adapted, it can be said that has entered the maintenance stage. Ambivalence will be present in all motivational stages, with relapse into the previous behavior always a possibility. This is why researchers have organized these stages in the form of a spiral, with every relapse being seen as a circling of the spiral, getting ever closer to the maintenance stage.

MI believes the process of change is the patient's responsibility, and depends on their performance. With this in mind, Miller and Rollnick (1991) defined five principles that underlie the motivational approach and provide the process of change. According to these principles, the therapist helps the patient carry out change in whatever stage of change they find themselves. The principles are as follows:

- Expressing empathy: empathy is the capacity to understand another's feelings and perspectives without judging, criticizing or blaming. The effect of empathy is that of making the patient feel understood and accepted, which leads them to achieve self-liberation and conceive of change. This acceptance that the therapist offers the patient also favors the forging of a good therapeutic alliance and builds the patient's self-esteem, which will be important in establishing change (Miller and Rollnick, 1991). It is essential that the motivational therapist consider ambivalence as something normal, both with regard to the human condition and to change itself. If a patient feels understood when going back and forth between wanting and not wanting change, this understanding itself can leverage their decision and make them change. In fact, ambivalence will be present in all the processes of change, and should be accepted and understood (Miller and Rollnick, 1991).
- Developing discrepancy: the therapist must point out the discrepancy between the patient's life goals and where their drinking and drug use behavior is leading them (Miller and Rollnick, 1991). According to Miller and Rollnick (1991), motivation for change comes when the individual perceives a discrepancy between their behaviors and the life goals they have defined. MI's main point is making the patient notice the reasons for change on their own. In general, people tend to value their own evaluation of the facts more than what others tell them. Therefore, in this approach, it is the patient who brings up their concerns, not the therapist (Miller and Rollnick, 1991).
- -Avoiding argument: It's essential that the psychotherapist avoid argument and direct confrontation with patients. Most of the time, patients start treatment conflicted, at the same time wanting and not wanting to change. This way, if the therapist argues in favor of change, the patient might strongly defend the opposite, and tend to remain as they are (Miller and Rollnick, 1991).
- -Rolling with resistance: it is the patient who must perceive their excessive drinking and drug use behavior as harmful, and the therapist's role is to promote this perception without pushing the patient. In order to do so, the therapist tries to alter the perceptions that make the patient resistant to change, encouraging them to consider other aspects of their actions. The decision to change always comes from the individual. Therefore, the therapist cannot persuade the patient nor show them solutions, instead assisting them in coming up with their own solutions (Miller and Rollnick, 1991).
- - Supporting Self-Efficacy: this involves the patient's hope and capacity to carry out change. In promoting self-efficacy, the therapist builds the individual's confidence in their own ability to handle a task or challenge. (Miller and Rollnick, 1991).

4.2 Cognitive model

Beck et al (1993) developed a cognitive model specifically to address the problem of substance abuse. People who present drug and alcohol problems tend to have core and intermediate beliefs regarding lack of love, helplessness, hopelessness and a low threshold for frustration and boredom. Intermediate beliefs are referred to as addictive beliefs and can be separated into other categories, forming a belief scheme.

When someone starts using a substance, anticipatory beliefs appear. At first, these beliefs take the form of statements such as "drinking will make me feel better" or "it's ok to use every now and then". As the person starts obtaining gratification from the drug, beliefs start changing into statements such as "smoking relaxes me" or "drinking makes me more cheerful". Anticipatory beliefs change according to the "anticipation → use → anticipation dysphoria → use" cycle into relief-oriented beliefs, and from these to permissive beliefs (Beck et al., 1993).

When permissive beliefs appear, beliefs that are contrary to use develop concomitantly, especially with regard to illegal drugs. These are called control beliefs. Permissive beliefs and control beliefs manifest simultaneously in the subject, and using or refraining from using drugs is a result of the conflict between permissive and control beliefs (Beck et al., 1993).

Activation of permissive beliefs occurs in the presence of certain activating stimuli, those that can activate the person's cravings and beliefs regarding use. These situations are individual and may vary in degree of risk. A situation can be very activating one day and not present any risk to the subject on another day or another time (Beck et al., 1993).

The cognitive model for substance abuse was organized in the following manner:

$$\text{Activating stimuli} \rightarrow \text{activating beliefs} \rightarrow \text{AT} \rightarrow \text{craving}$$

$$\uparrow \qquad\qquad\qquad\qquad\qquad\qquad\qquad\qquad \downarrow$$

$$\text{continue using} \leftarrow \text{instrumental strategies} \leftarrow \text{facilitating beliefs}$$

Cognitive therapy works on each of the belief categories: anticipatory, permissive and core. The therapist will introduce or reinforce better adaptive beliefs. The cognitive-behavioral therapist helps the patient act based on more realistic thoughts regarding their problem. Upon restructuring their thoughts, the subject starts to take charge of problems and situations previously considered unbearable, and that many times led them to use or abuse a substance (Beck et al., 1993).

4.3 Relapse prevention

The goal of relapse prevention (RP) is to prevent or limit the occurrence of relapse based on a combination of behavioral abilities and cognitive interventions (Marlatt and Donovan, 2005). The core factor in this approach is the view of addictive behaviors as hyper-learned and maladaptive habits. In many cases, people present maladaptive coping mechanisms when faced with stressful situations (for instance, smoking or drinking to reduce anxiety). It should be noted that the individual is not responsible for their acquired habit, nor are they in voluntary control of the behavior. However, the individual takes active responsibility during the process of habit change (Marlatt and Gordon, 1999).

Some factors are considered vital in approaching addictive behaviors:

- Determinants of addictive behaviors, including situational and environmental history, beliefs and expectations, individual history, and previous learning experiences with psychoactive substances or activities.

• The consequences of behaviors whose goal is to better understand both the reinforcing effects that may increase use and the negative consequences that may serve to inhibit use. In addition to the effects of drugs on activities, attention is paid to social and interpersonal relationships experienced by the individual before, during and after engaging in addictive behavior. Social factors are involved in social learning of the addictive behavior, as well as in the subsequent performance of those activities.

Relapse is seen as a transactional process, as a series of events that may or may not lead the person back to the initial pattern of behavior, the same pattern they had before contemplating a change directed at quitting or cutting down on substance use. The return to the previous pattern of behavior is called a relapse, and substance use following the return to the change process is called a lapse. One of the main goals of the treatment is to teach the patient to keep substance use during the change process in a state of lapse, so that it won't evolve into a state of relapse (Marlatt and Gordon, 1999).

When the subject falls into the latter state, relapse can also serve to provide information on what caused the event, and, this way, find ways to correct the problem so as to avoid new relapses. In this case, Marlatt and Gordon (1999) refer to such an event as a prolapse, as it places the individual in an advanced stage.

It is also important to discover determinants and common reactions to the first lapse, and to understand how these factors affect the likelihood of relapse or recovery. Furthermore, RP does not ignore the fact that each substance has particular characteristics and activities that influence use/abuse (Marlatt and Gordon, 1985).

Marlatt and Gordon (1985) initially presented the following relapse model:

Relapse response   →   ↑self-efficacy   →   ↓ relapse likelihood

↑

High-risk situation

↓

No coping → ↓ self-efficacy / expectations → early use → EVA → ↑ relapse likelihood
response   with respect to substance
                             positive result

In order to understand the scheme, it is assumed that the subject presents a perceived control or self-efficacy during the abstinence period. Thus, the better self-efficacy is perceived, the longer the abstinence period. The person will remain abstinent until a high-risk situation occurs, at which point their sense of control increases the risk of relapse.

The three most common types of relapse factors are negative emotional states, interpersonal conflicts, and social pressure. Negative emotional states correspond to situations in which the individual experiences a negative mood, feeling or emotional state at the moment when lapse occurs, such as, for instance, anger, sadness, anxiety, boredom, etc. Interpersonal conflicts involve an ongoing or recent conflict associated to any interpersonal relationship. The social pressure factor corresponds to situations in which the person is suffering influence from another person or group that exerts pressure, leading to the undesired behavior.

According to the scheme, after the risk situation, the individual will follow one of two paths. One is that of carrying out an effective behavioral or cognitive coping response. When someone is successful in one situation, the likelihood increases that they will be successful in the next situation with which they are faced. The feeling of confidence in one's own ability is related to self-efficacy, and so the more one faces high-risk situations successfully, the lower the likelihood of a relapse.

The other path a person may take after being faced with a high-risk situation occurs because they may not have acquired coping abilities, or the appropriate response may have been inhibited by fear or anxiety. Another possibility is that the person may not have perceived the situation as a high-risk one. This leads to a decrease in self-efficacy, a feeling of impotence and a tendency towards apathy. If the person is also tempted to use the substance, there is increased probability of a relapse. The probability is even higher when the individual has maintained positive expectations regarding the effects of the substance. Therefore, the inability to cope with high-risk situations, along with the expectations of positive results, greatly increase the probability that a lapse will occur. All this leads to a decrease in self-efficacy. Whether or not this first lapse will signify a total relapse will depend on the person's perceptions of the cause of the lapse and the reactions associated to the event.

RP does not see abstinence from an "all or nothing" perspective, and works with a mechanism called Violation Effect (AVE). AVE occurs in certain circumstances, such as before the first lapse, when the individual is personally committed to an extended or indefinite abstinence period. Furthermore, there are factors that may interfere in the AVE intensity, such as severe external justification, commitment strength or the effort made to maintain abstinence, the presence of key people, perception of the lapse as voluntary or as a preplanned activity, the value or importance of the undesirable behavior, among others. There is also the hypothesis that AVE can be intensified by affective cognitive elements, such as cognitive dissonance (conflict and guilt) and the effect of personal attribution (blaming oneself for the relapse).

Another effect of AVE is attributing the cause of the lapse to personal weakness or failure. In sum, AVE proposes a way to see lapses that is not an "all or nothing" process. According to AVE, the person can avoid the lapse through a combination of greater awareness, coping abilities, accepting responsibility, and personal choice.

Later on, Witkiewitz and Marlatt (2004) proposed some changes to this model when they concluded that the relapse process was more complex than previously thought. They proposed the dynamic relapse model. In this model, relapse determinants are seen as multidimensional and dynamic. Each risk situation the patient faces sets off triggers and their consequences. The person's response is complex, involving distal risk factors, cognitive processes and cognitive-behavioral coping abilities. Distal risk factors are, for instance, family history, substance consumption time, social life, and co-morbid psychopathology. Cognitive processes involve self-efficacy, result expectations, craving, AVE, and motivation (Marlatt and Donovan, 2005). Distal risks, cognitive processes and coping ability can interact in various ways, and there is a cause-and-effect relationship between them, that is, they may end up influencing one another (Marlatt and Donovan, 2005).

4.4 Most commonly used techniques

4.4.1 Reflective listening

Simple reflection. This technique consists of offering a sentence or part of a sentence back to the speaker. It is important that the sentence be offered back in the form of an assertion, rather than a question. The goal is for the patient to reflect on what they are saying. It's a good strategy to be used when the patient is resistant to behavior change, as well as a way for the therapist to show understanding and acceptance.

Amplified reflection. This technique is used to reflect something the patient said in an exaggerated and amplified manner. At this point, the psychotherapist makes an assertion in a more exaggerated tone than the one used by the patient. If well carried out, amplified reflection will encourage the patient to take a step back and give change some thought. One must be cautious about the tone of voice used, as a sarcastic tone may elicit a hostile and resistant reaction. Radical terms, such as "never", "always", "all", and "nothing" should be avoided in this reflection.

Double-sided reflection. This reflection technique consists of acknowledging what the patient said and adding the other side of the ambivalence, based on the material the patient had already put forth in a previous moment. An example of double-sided reflection would be, "On the one hand, you acknowledge the harmfulness of drinking; on the other hand, drinking with your friends is your only time to relax."

Paraphrasing. The goal of this technique is to paraphrase the information that the patient himself/herself brings. This technique is used mainly when the patient puts forth arguments for denying the social problem. In paraphrasing, the therapist acknowledges what the patient says and offers a new meaning or interpretation. Just as reflections, paraphrasing must always be an assertion, never a question.

4.4.2 Pros and cons

This involves having the patient write down, in an objective manner, the pros and cons of using and not using the substance. A 2 x 2 matrix is then built so that the four squares can help the patient to better visualize their options, as they're able to analyze each of the pros and cons.

4.4.3 Coping cards

These are cards of a portable size that the patient can carry anywhere they go. On these cards, notes are written down which, in risk situations, will help them resist a relapse. The patient chooses the notes that will be most helpful in facing said situations, but these are some examples: pros and cons, distraction techniques, and breathing exercises.

4.4.4 Self-monitoring

This involves making a daily or weekly record of substance consumption. In these records, the patient describes the number of occasions and time of day in which they use, and may also include thoughts and feelings associated to the activity. This technique allows the patient to become aware of the dimension their problem has reached and how present it is in their life. For this reason, it's a technique that is used mainly when beginning treatment. It may be used during sessions by asking the patient for an account of a typical day when the substance is consumed, or it can be assigned as homework, so that the patient can record the instances of consumption as they occur throughout the week.

4.4.5 Identifying and restructuring automatic thoughts

The patient learns to identify thoughts that generate the desire to drink or use the drug, as well as those that keep them active while the patient continues to use the substance. Once thoughts are identified, they can be restructured, that is, the patient learns how to interpret the situation so as to weaken the desire to use the substance or to engage in any harmful behavior.

4.4.6 Problem solving

Escaping from problems is a very common reason for people to engage in drug and alcohol abuse. Because of this, the problem solving technique is important in helping patients imagine and find an efficient solution to a problem. This can be done in six steps: (1) define the problem in a clear and specific way; (2) imagine as many solutions as possible through brainstorming; (3) examine the pros and cons of each selected solution, assessing their present and future consequences; (4) choose the best hypothetical solution; (5) implement the chosen solution through planning, preparation, and practice; (6) evaluate success and, in case the problem is not solved, return to step 4.

4.4.7 Social skills training

Consists of capacitating the patient to respond in an effective and adequate way to certain situations that may put them at risk or that are already a risk, such as, for instance, being invited to a bar. This training must contain strategies with which the patient can avoid or abandon a risk situation, and should explore the patient's family, social, and work environments. During training, the patient's level of anxiety must be evaluated and is expected to decrease as adequate behaviors are maintained.

4.4.8 Craving management

This consists of learning awareness of craving for alcohol or drugs and understanding its components. Based on this, a way of managing these symptoms is offered through techniques involving distraction, relaxation, problem solving, ability training and coping cards (notes to help patients deal with risk situations).

4.4.9 Distraction

The main goal of distraction techniques is to change the patient's focus from their inner world (thoughts, memories, physical symptoms) to the outer environment. This technique is very useful in moments of craving, when patients are at risk for a relapse. According to Beck et al. (1993) there are some resources that can be easily employed which enable the patient to find a distraction:

1. Patients are instructed to focus their attention on what is around them, such as the landscape, people, cars, furniture, etc.
2. Talking to other people. This may involve initiating conversation, calling a friend or even joining a group.
3. Leaving the place they find themselves in. Visiting a friend, driving or going to the supermarket, for instance.
4. Carrying out domestic chores, such as doing dishes, organizing closets or fixing appliances. In addition to distracting the person, these activities build self-esteem, since they'll be doing something useful.
5. Reciting a favorite poem or prayer, or even writing them down.
6. Engaging in recreational activities, such as attention-demanding games: videogames, cards, puzzles, crossword puzzles.

Example of an Intervention

The identification of factors and the skills to deal with them was developed in a group treatment consisting of 27 ninety-minute sessions held twice a week for patients referred by the Worker Health Inspection Division (DVST) of the Federal University of Rio de Janeiro to the Alcoholism Rehabilitation and Research Center (now the Teaching, Research and Reference Center for Alcohology and Addictology – CEPRAL). The goal was to develop a treatment program for alcohol addicts based on a cognitive-behavioral approach whose aim would be early full remission.

The specific goals were: (1) to develop learning and practice of new behaviors to replace the drinking behavior through training in intrapersonal and interpersonal skills; (2) to teach coping strategies to be used when dealing with internal and external high-risk situations that could trigger addictive behavior; (3) to establish general strategies for modifying one's lifestyle, and (4) to develop strategies that would favor adherence to the process of change produced by the treatment.

Interpersonal skills training involved learning to recognize social signs, developing the ability to initiate, maintain and redirect conversations with strangers and acquaintances, strengthening assertive behaviors, such as saying "no" or requesting that others change their behavior. Intrapersonal skills were related to learning muscle and/or breathing relaxation strategies, anger management, and cognitive restructuring to reduce states of anxiety and/or depressive moods. Other skills that were considered important included identifying high-risk situations for relapse, such as going to bar on a Friday night while depressed and abstinent for several days, as well as facilitating beliefs that can lead to alcohol use. Strategies for lifestyle changes included actions that encourage an increase in activity, especially enjoyable activities, as well as motivation to take part in new social groups.

The working hypotheses were that training in social skills would be efficient in treating alcoholism, with the end goal being alcohol consumption abstinence, defined as Early Full Remission in the DSM-IV (APA, 2002); that addictive behavior is functionally related to deficits in skills for coping with everyday problem situations, and that acquiring skills for recognizing and handling risk situations contributes to adherence to a state of Early Full Remission.

Some of the instruments used included anamnesis interview, Structured Interview for Anxiety Disorders for DSM-IV (ADIS-4), Structured Interview for Personality Disorders for DSM-IV (SCID-TP), Beck Anxiety and Depression Inventories, Hamilton Anxiety Inventories (HAMA) and (HAMD). The results of these inventories were compared to applications at the end of the program.

Below is a description of a hypothetical group intervention for other groups.

A first session can include introduction to the work plan, the rules and norms that will guide the work within the group, and introduction of each of the members, including a brief report of their problem for evaluation. The goals can be making patients feel comfortable, having them interact with one another and receive orientation regarding the group's general principles, goals, procedures, and rules. The relapse prevention model, cognitive model, and social skills training model can also be introduced.

The second session can be dedicated to handling alcohol-related thoughts, encouraging members to replace thoughts of drinking with other thoughts by means of group discussion and exercises. A list of pros and cons with regard to drinking behavior can be made so as to make the benefits of not drinking clearer when compared to drinking. This list would be based on the members' past experiences with alcohol.

The third session can be dedicated to developing problem solving strategies – acknowledging that problems exist, but can be solved. The first step is knowing how to identify the problem. This is followed by a brainstorming session in which several different solutions, even those that could be considered strange, are presented. After that, the pros and cons of each one are objectively analyzed, a hierarchy is established, and the most promising alternative is used. If this alternative works and solves the problem, then good; if not, the next one is used, and so on. Role-playing and discussion techniques may be used with the group.

Subsequent sessions can be dedicated to social skills training, aiming for establishing a conversation with the goal of developing basic communication skills, based on the idea that conversation is the first step in establishing interpersonal relationships. In order to make starting a conversation easier, it is suggested that open questions be used so as to encourage a response. This type of question always includes the use of adverbs such as *when, since when, where, what, how, why,* etc. The reply will be longer and this may favor identification of any common experiences. These communication techniques also recommend that the person speak about themselves, describing facts and experiences, since this increases chances of finding something in common with the other person. It is very important to emphasize the development of listening and observation skills. The conversation may be ended politely, leaving the other with the feeling that the conversation was pleasant. Obstacles that may make it difficult for each of the members to establish effective communication must be identified so that they can be overcome.

The session in which assertiveness training will start will be held after basic social skills have been strengthened. These skills require learning to express feelings in a direct, honest, and adequate manner, speaking in a clear, firm, and decisive tone, establishing eye contact, using "me" statements ("I prefer it when you act this way toward me", "I don't appreciate your yelling at me", etc). Through role-playing, debates, and exercises, members of the group learn to say "no" and suggest alternatives. They can also learn to request that other people change their behavior in cases where these people are insistent in their invitations to go drinking. Other sessions on this topic can be dedicated to making and receiving compliments, offering and taking criticism, refusing alcoholic beverages, and so on.

Subsequent sessions can be dedicated to close personal relationships, aiming at developing skills to deal with the difficulties and conflicts that appear in the context of such relationships. In order to establish effective communication, it's very important to combine skills such as being assertive, showing an ability to express positive feelings, offering and taking constructive criticism regarding upsetting behaviors before negative feelings can accumulate, making and receiving compliments, and listening actively. Being a dynamic listener helps build proximity, affection, support, and understanding. It's also important to have direct conversations with one's partner about sex, so that they can become aware of what you think, feel, and want. Special emphasis should be given to certain relationship skills, such as expressing feelings in an empathetic and assertive manner, ability to discuss and negotiate, solving problems and conflicts, personal change, and helping the other change. Generalizing and transferring this knowledge to everyday life will depend on each person's comprehension and consistent training for reaching this goal.

The importance of non-verbal communication must be emphasized to the extent that there needs to be a correspondence between verbal behavior (what is said) and non-verbal behavior (how it is said). This is done by discussing the different components of non-verbal communication: posture, space (distance) between people, eye contact, head signals, facial expression, tone of voice, gestures and miming. Role-playing can be used to model these exercises.

Breathing and muscle relaxation exercises, as well as imagination techniques, should be introduced, seeing as many drinkers use alcohol as a sort of self-medication to help them relax and control tension, stress, and anxiety. It is important to learn to be aware of tension in the body, and to learn how to relax by tensing and relaxing eight specific muscle groups. This progressive muscle relaxation was conceived by Jacobson (1938) and has been widely used in CBT since the 1950s (Conrad & Roth, 2007). Relaxation exercises can be carried out in groups, combining suggestive techniques taken from autogenic training (Schultz, 1967) and imaginary technique exercises with positive visualization. Another kind of relaxation that can be used during these sessions are breathing technique exercises, described as diaphragmatic breathing, such as those used in yoga and/or meditation classes.

Regarding the learning of intrapersonal techniques, the first one can be dedicated to anger management, since anger is the main factor related to relapses. Therefore, learning to discriminate anger triggers and knowing how to function under the effect of this emotion is very important, hence the need to define anger and highlight its positive and negative effects. It's essential to differentiate situations that trigger anger directly or indirectly, as well as the responses they manifest (internal reactions). Another very important point to highlight is that anger, like all emotions, has a duration, and that it necessarily decreases and passes. For this reason, firstly it must be pointed out that the first thing a person can do when feeling angry is do *nothing*. Secondly, the person should start diaphragmatic breathing. Thirdly, they should reflect on the interpretation they've made of the event that may have triggered anger in order to check if their assessment is correct, if there have been distortions, or if other interpretations can be conceived of. Finally, if they have calmed down, the person can start talking in an assertive manner to the one whose behavior triggered the anger. It's a good idea to examine situations that cause the group members to get angry, and to use stress inoculation exercises in order to help them learn anger management.

Sessions can also be dedicated to obtaining a reversal of negative thoughts. Learning to identify negative or pessimistic thoughts is important for changing them and being able to notice how they influence our feelings. Learning to restructure them and replace them with other, more realistic thoughts is useful and necessary if one wants to do away with feelings of sadness, which are another source of relapses. This skill can be incorporated through practical exercises using record forms for dysfunctional thoughts and group role-playing. More specifically, it may be necessary to try to change core beliefs that are irrational and unrealistic, and replace them with more realistic beliefs.

Further on, a revision can be made of relapse prevention and cognitive models (beliefs and automatic thoughts), social skills training (assertiveness, non-verbal behavior, offering and taking criticism, negotiating), and the importance of empathy in close personal relationships. Relaxation training and problem solving training can be redone. Further attention should be paid to coping with feelings such as anger, fear, tension, sadness, and joy.

Increasing time spent on enjoyable activities with the goal of highlighting the importance of the amount of time dedicated to leisure and enjoyable activities is a way of avoiding negative thoughts. Patients should try to develop a variety of enjoyable activities through the enjoyment chart technique (Rangé, 1995) and a wish list, highlighting the identification of obstacles. Increasing the social support network is a necessary goal for developing and maintaining interpersonal relationships that can provide the support a person needs to feel more confident in their abilities. It is also important to identify ways in which interactions can be a source of support: (1) who can provide help? (2) what kind of support is sought? (3) how can you obtain the help you need? Finally, it is necessary to demonstrate, with the goal of obtaining a model, effective ways (direct and specific requests) and ineffective ways (indirect, unspecific requests) to ask for support.

Is it also essential to dedicate attention to emergency plans for a variety of stressful situations that can arise unexpectedly, and include strategies for solving them. It is also necessary to deal with persistent problems, taking into account the changes that have occurred since the treatment began and identifying the problems that still persist.

The last session is again dedicated to a conversation about relapse prevention, considering the increase in awareness that apparently irrelevant decisions can help trigger relapses. It's important to highlight the ability to think about each choice, anticipate risks, and analyze the last relapses and the apparently irrelevant decisions that may have led to them. An analysis of the treatment is made, including patient feedback, so that the group can be properly dismissed.

5. Conclusions

Working with individuals who have drug and/or alcohol abuse issues is not usually very gratifying, but maybe it is stimulating precisely due to this. In dealing with patients who are addicts, it is important that the therapist remain "centered", trying not to demonstrate helplessness or hopelessness, while at the same time not expecting constant progress. The therapist must provide his or her patient with feedback, training, techniques, and support, but, at the same time the therapist cannot accept responsibility for the patient's problems. The therapist must always remain calm in the face of a crisis situation and help the patient apply problem solving, while knowing that he or she cannot solve crises for them.

6. References

American Psychiatric Association. Manual Diagnóstico e Estatístico de Transtornos Mentais. 4 ed. Texto revisado (–DSM-IV-TR). Porto Alegre: Artmed; 2002

Beck A.T.; Wright, F.; Newman,C.; Liese,B. (1993) Cognitive Therapy of Substance Abuse. New York: The Guilford Press.

Bolton J, Cox B, Clara I, Sareen J. Use of alcohol and drugs to self-medicate anxiety disorders in a nationally representative sample. J Nerv Ment Dis. 2006 Nov;194(11):818-25.

Ferron JC, Brunette MF, He X, Xie H, McHugo GJ, Drake RE. Course of smoking and quit attempts among clients with co-occurring severe mental illness and substance use disorders. Psychiatr Serv. 2011 Apr;62(4):353-9.

Ilgen MA, Hu KU, Moos RH, McKellar J. Continuing care after inpatient psychiatric treatment for patients with psychiatric and substance use disorders. Psychiatr Serv. 2008 Sep;59(9):982-8.

Marlatt, G.A. Donovan, D.M. (2005). Relapse Prevention: maintenance strategies in the treatment of addictive behaviors. New York: Guilford Press.

Marlatt, G.A. Gordon, J.R. (1985). Relapse Prevention. Guilford Press.

Mathias, A.C.R., Vargens, R.W., Kessler, F.H., Cruz, M.S. Differences in Addiction Severity Between Social and Probable Pathological Gamblers Among Substance Abusers in Treatment in Rio de Janeiro. Int J Ment Health Addiction. 2009, 9: 239-249.

Miller W.R. & Rollnick, S. (1991). Motivational interviewing: Preparing people to change addictive behavior. New York: Guilford Press.

Monti P.M., Kadden, R.M., Rohsenow, D.J., Cooney, N.L., Abrams, D.B. (2005) Tratando a Dependência de Álcool: Um Guia de Treinamento das Habilidades de Enfrentamento (seg. ed.). São Paulo: Roca.

Rosenheck R, Desai R. Substance use comorbidity among veterans with posttraumatic stress disorder and other psychiatric illness. Am J Addict. 2011 May-Jun;20(3):185-9.

Prochaska, J. O., & DiClemente, C. C. (1982). Transtheoretical therapy Toward a more integrative model of change. Psychotherapy: Theory, research and practice, 19, 276-288.

Substance Abuse and Mental Health Services Administration (2009) Results from the 2008 National Survey on Drug Use and Health: National Findings (Office of Applied Studies, NSDUH Series H-36, HHS Publication No. SMA 09-4434). Rockville, MD.

Robinson J, Sareen J, Cox BJ, Bolton JM. Role of Self-medication in the Development of Comorbid Anxiety and Substance Use Disorders: A Longitudinal Investigation. Arch Gen Psychiatry. 2011 Aug;68(8):800-7.

Swendsen J, Conway KP, Degenhardt L, Glantz M, Jin R, Merikangas KR, Sampson N, Kessler RC. Mental disorders as risk factors for substance use, abuse and dependence: results from the 10-year follow-up of the National Comorbidity Survey. Addiction. 2010 Jun;105(6):1117-28.

Vijayakumar L, Kumar MS, Vijayakumar V. Substance use and suicide. Curr Opin Psychiatry. 2011 May;24(3):197-202.

Witkiewitz, K. Marlatt, G.A. (2004) Relapse prevention for alcohol and drug problems: That was zen, this is tao. American Psychologist, 59, 224-235.

9

A Proposed Learning Model
of Body Dysmorphic Disorder

Fugen Neziroglu and Lauren M. Mancusi
Bio-Behavioral Institute, Great Neck, NY
USA

1. Introduction

While it is common for individuals to have concerns about their appearance, individuals with body dysmorphic disorder (BDD) experience a marked distress that often results in time-consuming rituals, social anxiety, and depression among other debilitating effects. Body dysmorphic disorder (BDD) is a severe and debilitating disorder that is characterized by a perceived physical defect that causes significant impairments in everyday functioning (American Psychiatric Association, 2000). BDD was first mention in the late 1800's (Morselli, 1891). It was described as dysmorphophobia and referred to a strong emotional response (e.g. anxiety) to certain changes in physical appearance. Body dysmorphic disorder was not mentioned again until the advent of the third *Diagnostic and Statistical Manual for Mental Disorders* (DSM III), in which BDD was listed as a somotaform disorder (American Psychiatric Association, 1987). While BDD remains classified as a somotaform disorder in the current edition of the DSM (DSM IV-TR), more recently it has been conceptualized as an obsessive-compulsive related disorder (OCRD). Like other OCRD, BDD involves symptoms of obsessions and compulsions.

Similar to obsessive compulsive disorder (OCD), individuals with BDD experience intrusive thoughts and/or images. The obsessive nature of BDD is usually centered around a perceived, or slight defect in physical appearance. The BDD concern can be general (e.g. an overall feeling of ugliness or feeling too feminine or masculine) or focus on a specific feature. The most common preoccupations are around the face, particularly the nose, skin, hair, eyes, mouth, lips, jaw, and chin. However, the preoccupation can focus on any body part and often involves several body parts. Additionally, the location of the main flaw or defect can change over time (Veale & Neziroglu, 2010).

The preoccupation greatly impairs one's social, occupational, and/or academic functioning (American Psychiatric Association, 2000), and typically leads to compulsive behaviors in an attempt to decrease the anxiety and distress experienced. Common compulsions include safety and/or avoidance behaviors such as mirror-checking, mirror-avoidance, camouflaging, excessive grooming, reassurance seeking, and skin picking.

The level of dysfunction caused by BDD symptoms is very disabling. Individuals with BDD have poor employment history, low marital rates, higher suicide rates than the general population, and typically present with high degrees of co-morbid mood disorders (Neziroglu, Khemlani-Patel, & Jacofsky, 2009; Phillips & Menard, 2006). Gunstand and

Phillips (2003) examined rates of depression in 293 individuals with BDD. They found 59% of participants at the time of the study had major depression and a lifetime rate of depression of 76%. Moreover, individuals with BDD experience an array of negative emotions including anxiety and shame. Many individuals with BDD often do not seek medical and/or psychological treatment due to their experience of shame and self disgust. They do not want to be perceived as vain or superficial. Initially, many seek alternative treatments for their perceived defect such as dermatological procedures and cosmetic surgery. Often, when individuals with BDD seek psychological treatment it is for a co-morbid condition. In fact, many BDD patients do not typically present for treatment until 10-15 years after the age of symptom onset (McKay & Neziroglu, 2011). By the time they enter into treatment, their BDD concern is strengthened and maintained and can be very challenging to treat.

The lapse of time between symptom onset and entering into treatment makes it difficult to formulate a comprehensive etiology of the disorder because most of what is known is based on patient reports. Although the etiology of BDD is unknown, various models attempt to explain the disorder. Models are structures or frameworks based on hypotheses that explain how a certain disorder develops, progresses, and is maintained. Models guide research aimed at developing efficacious treatments (Neziroglu et al., 2009; Rabinowitz, Neziroglu, & Khemlani-Patel, 2007). Current models of BDD include aesthetic sensitivity and the self as an aesthetic object (Veale, Ennis, Lambrou, 2002), social learning and conditioning (Neziroglu, Khemlani-Patel, & Veale, 2008), neurobiological (Yaryura-Tobias, Neziroglu, Chang, et al., 2002; Yaryura-Tobias, Neziroglu & Torres-Gallegos, 2002; Saxena & Feusner, 2006; , Feusner, Townsend, Bystritsky & Bookheimer, 2007; Feusner, Yaryura-Tobias, & Saxena, 2008,), and neuroanatomical (Rauch, Phillips, Segal, Makris, Shin, Whalen,et al., 2003).

The learning model by Neziroglu and colleagues (Neziroglu, Khemlani-Patel, & Veale, 2008; Neziroglu, Robert, & Yaryura-Tobias, 2004) is similar to Cash's (2002) general CBT model of body image disturbance. This model proposes that cultural socialization, interpersonal experiences, physical characteristics, and personality attributes contribute to the development of body image perception and attitudes (e.g. body satisfaction). The importance and/or sensitivity about attractiveness significantly contribute to the beliefs, assumptions, and values that are developed in individuals with BDD (Wilhelm & Neziroglu, 2002).

The key components of the CBT model for BDD are shown in Figure 1 and include a) a biological predisposition; b) initial operant conditioning; c) social and/or vicarious learning; d) classical/evaluative conditioning; e) relational responding; and f) secondary operant conditioning (Neziroglu et al., 2008; Neziroglu, Roberts, & Yaryura-Tobias, 2004).

2. Cognitive behavioral model of body dysmorphic disorder

2.1 Biological predisposition

The proposed learning model of BDD keeps with the diathesis-stress model concerning mental disorders suggests that some individuals are genetically predisposed to develop a psychological disorder in times of stress. A biological predisposition alone does not necessarily predict whether one will develop a specific disorder. Rather, the development of BDD, or any psychological disorder, is the result of an interaction of a variety of factors, including a biological predisposition. Biological predispositions include genetic factors, visual processing problems, somatosensory problems, and changes in neuroanatomical/neurochemical circuitry (Neziroglu et al., 2004).

2.2 Initial operant conditioning

The CBT model of BDD hypothesizes that operant conditioning coupled with social learning results in the development of values and beliefs about attractiveness, as well as a sense of the self's value being conditionally based on body image (Neziroglu et al., 2004). Childhood experiences that positively reinforce an individual for appearance can contribute to BDD development. These experiences may reinforce the notion that appearance is important despite the accompanying behavior (e.g. comments such as "You looked so beautiful in your dance costume!" rather than "You danced so beautifully in your recital"). While many individuals with BDD were not positively or intermittently reinforced for their overall appearance, many were reinforced as children or adolescents for certain parts of their appearance such as, height, weight, body shape, and poise. Individuals with BDD report general childhood and adolescent experiences where their appearance was valued and exaggerated such as being in the attractive crowd in school or early dating success.

While positive reinforcement for appearance plays an important role in BDD development, early childhood and adolescent experiences need not be positive to have an influence. Negative experiences (e.g. teasing, bullying, and neglect) may prepare an individual for the negative affect s/he feels when observing body parts later in life (Osman, Cooper, Hackmann, & Veale, 2004; Phillips, 1996a). These experiences may become part of the core beliefs concerning the value of attractiveness.

2.3 Social and/or vicarious learning

Social and/or vicarious learning occurs when others are observed being rewarded or punished for a particular belief or behavior (Bandura, 1977). An individual may learn or strengthen beliefs by learning how others are rewarded. From an early age, individuals learn that physical attractiveness yields rewards. The association between self worth and physical attractiveness is reinforced by observed experiences in which other attractive individuals are positively reinforced and by society's overvaluation of physical attractiveness (Rabinowitz et al., 2007). This is extremely salient in the media and popular culture. Most, if not all, leading television and movie roles are played by attractive men and women. Children and adolescents are taught that physical attractiveness is necessary for success. Furthermore, television commercials and magazines advertise a multitude of cosmetic products to help achieve the goal of beauty.

In addition to the bombarding images in the media, vicarious learning extends beyond the sociocultural environment to one's immediate environment. Family members can express over concern about their own appearance and extend this preoccupation to their children, making frequent comments about their child's appearance. This further confirms that appearance is an important factor that is valued in society.

2.4 Symptom development through classical and evaluative conditioning

BDD development is formulated to be a function of classical (conditioning of liking or disliking of stimuli) or evaluative conditioning (conditioning of physiological responses). In the case of BDD, negative events about one's physical appearance may serve as the unconditioned stimulus (UCS) (e.g. being teased about reaching puberty early) and cause an unconditioned emotional response (UCR) (e.g. anxiety, depression, disgust, or shame). The unconditioned stimulus (UCS) is evaluated as negative and therefore, anything paired with it is evaluated as negative as well. For example, a person is teased (UCS) for having a big nose and this evokes a negative affect. Subsequently, a word (CS: "big") or a body part (CS: "nose") is evaluated as negative. According to evaluative conditioning, any previously neutral body part or word ("big") can take on the same negative reaction as the UCS. When an individual is exposed to the body part of concern, a negative emotional response is elicited. Not only is the CS evaluated negatively, but it evokes the same response as the UCS (e.g. anxiety, shame, or disgust).

2.4.1 Information processing/development of belief system based on relational frame theory

Early experiences and conditioning begin to shape an individual's cognitions and emotions. However, human beings have the capacity for language. Language mediates conditioning and learning in humans and significantly contributes to the strengthening and development of appearance related beliefs. Relational frame theory explains the role of language and how it influences emotions and cognitions (Hayes, Barnes-Holmes, & Roche, 2001). Three of the main premises of relational frame theory and how they relate to BDD are highlighted below.

2.4.2 Bi-directional stimulus relations

Only for humans, does a word and the actual item or event enter into a bi-directional stimulus relation, wherein each can equally stand for the other (e.g. the words "potato chip" and the actual potato chip are equal). Because of our capacity for language, we do not need to see the potato chip to anticipate having one. Hearing "potato chip" is a powerful enough stimulus, and the words "potato chip" and the actual potato chip are equally powerful reinforcers. Our ability to use language allows us to learn about things and events even if we have never experienced the particular event. Furthermore, for animals, order in which the words "potato chip" is said and the actual potato chip is presented is important. However, for children the order of the words and presentation of the actual item does not matter. The words "potato chip" could be said either before or after a child eats the potato chip. Once the child learns the words "potato chip", other similar reinforcers can be taught, so that both elicit the thought even though the child may not have had direct experience with the second stimulus. For example, we can teach a child that a "potato chip" is similar to a "pretzel" and eventually both words, "potato chip" and "pretzel," will elicit the thought "potato chip" and "pretzel," even if the child has never seen a pretzel. This bi-directionality is the most important defining feature of human language and cognition. It explains why evaluative conditioning can occur and why arbitrary associations can be made.

2.4.3 Relational frames

The ability to think relationally allows us not only to make predictions, but allows our mind to generate various other relations. Language assists evaluative conditioning by stimulating complex networks of associated ideas, images, and evaluations. Relational responding occurs during early language by teaching relational frames (e.g. learning that things are "similar", learning temporal and causal relations – "before" and "after", "if..then," and comparative and evaluative – "bigger than, better than" etc.). Language assists classical conditioning. For example, a child could learn that having a scar (UCS) makes her feel disgust (UCR) and later, any scar (CS) elicits disgust (CR). Likewise, the words "cut," "scratch," or "wound" can elicit the same negative affect (classical/evaluative conditioning via relational frame of coordination or similarity). Words that connote similar concepts conjure up the same thoughts. This is why a BDD individual may respond with negative affect to any event or word that reminds him/her of a similar situation. If at some point a child had a disgust reaction to a scar, then anything similar to it can elicit the same reaction simply by thinking about it.

2.4.4 Arbitrary and non-arbitrary connections

Relational frame theory (Hayes et al., 2001) suggests that as human beings we use language as a way of making connections that may or may not be factual. Perhaps in the case of BDD, humans make arbitrary associations between appearance, social success, and/or undesirable human traits. For example, a child may hear an adult talking about a peer who whines incessantly. However, the adults may comment that the peer always looks beautiful and too bad, she is consistently whining. The child may learn that people will tolerate unpleasantness if the person is attractive, and therefore, beauty is important. Thus, people will accept unpleasant traits from attractive people. The child may begin to compare herself with her peer to see is she is just as pretty, in order for people to accept her as well.

In addition to language and cognitions, thoughts can take on meaning and elicit emotions. For example, if you think of a spoon you may have a neutral response, but if you think of a spoon that has fallen into the toilet bowl and later sanitized you may have a disgust reaction. This demonstrates that due to language, we make arbitrary associations and have certain emotional responses to those thoughts. There may be either direct conditioning of the CS and UCS occurring via the mediation of language. As the CS is paired with the CR, a set of cognitions is strengthened, information is processed, and a set of beliefs initially introduced through early life experiences continues to be reinforced. These beliefs may center on thoughts such as, "Being attractive is the most important thing in the world," "I can only succeed in life if I am attractive," "I am worthless if I am not attractive," etc. It is during this time that attention is drawn to the perceived defective body part. Selective attention to the defective part leads to more focused attention on the defect and thus, a strengthening of the conditioning process.

2.5 Higher order conditioning

Higher order conditioning may account for BDD symptoms secondary to the patient's primary concern (e.g. while mirror checking one body part, a secondary body part may become more noticeable and elicit the same negative response as the original area of concern). As a result of higher-order conditioning, the negative emotional reaction generalizes to other body parts that are noticed while evaluating the primary body part of concern (Neziroglu, et al., 2004).

Higher order conditioning may be direct or through relational framing. For example, children are taught to look at an object, then hear its name, and then say its name.

Eventually, children can hear the name and point to the object. Once the object-word and word-object relation is trained, relational responding occurs. If a child is taught, "This is your mouth, ear, and eye," then the child can identify the parts of the face when asked "Where is your mouth, ear, and eye?" even without differential reinforcement. This derived arbitrarily applicable relation is referred to as a "relational frame." It is brought under the control of contextual cues through a process of differential reinforcement. Once we, as human beings, are taught through reinforcement, we can generalize to novel situations without direct reinforcement by using what we have learned in the past. This is similar to higher-order conditioning where a CS is paired with another CS and therefore, generates the same response.

2.6 Maintenance of symptoms through operant conditioning

Once BDD appearance related beliefs, values, and assumptions are established, operant conditioning in the form of negative reinforcement maintains maladaptive cognitions and compulsions (Neziroglu et al., 2008; Neziroglu, et al., 2004). More specifically, compulsive behaviors serve to reduce short-term distress by "taking away" the negative emotional reaction triggered by either an intrusive thought or contact with the perceived flaw. Individuals with BDD engage in safety and/or avoidance behaviors such as mirror checking, mirror avoiding, camouflaging, excessive grooming, and/or reassurance-seeking in attempt to reduce the negative feelings such as anxiety, shame, and disgust (Neziroglu et al., 2008). BDD patients can be identified by two main types of compulsions: mirror checking or mirror avoiding. However, BDD patients can engage in both mirror checking and mirror avoiding behaviors. Those who engage in mirror checking may spend countless hours a day in front of a mirror scrutinizing their appearance and checking for flaws. They continuously attempt to fix their appearance to hide their flaw, so it is not noticeable to others. Those who engage in mirror avoiding go out of their way to avoid seeing their own reflection (e.g. covering/removing mirrors from their home, removing all reflective surfaces from their home) (Rabinowitz et al., 2007). For example, a BDD patient who engages in mirror avoidance experiences relief because of not being exposed to their image. This relief represents a negative reinforcer in that it allows one to avoid the anxiety associated with the perceived physical flaw thus, increasing the probability that the avoidance behavior will be used again when in a similar situation. Conversely, a BDD patient may engage in mirror checking and like the way he/she looks. In this case, the mirror checking behavior has decreased the anxiety associated with the perceived physical flaw. The random positive feedback encourages the patient to continue mirror checking. In either situation, the BDD patient's behavior has temporarily reduced the patient's anxiety concerning his or her appearance, and is maintained by negative reinforcement. Whether a BDD patient engages in mirror-checking, mirror-avoidance, camouflaging, or reassurance-seeking, each behavior aims at reducing the anxiety associated with the thoughts "Do I look horrible?" or "Has my appearance changed since I last looked at myself." Depending on the individual's mood state, expectations, lighting in the area, or mirror used different images may be perceived at different times. These variables may lead to more or less safety and/or avoidance behaviors. This is a variable- ratio schedule of reinforcement. Since variable ratios are the most successful schedules of reinforcement at increasing and maintaining behavior, the BDD behaviors are strong and thus, difficult to extinguish and treat.

3. Treatment approach derived from the model

Exposure and response prevention (ERP) is the preferred treatment for BDD. ERP applies basic behavioral principles such as habituation and extinction to reverse learning that has happened through classical and operant conditioning. In the case of BDD, ERP involves repeated exposures of the defective body part (CS) across multiple situations that elicit negative responses (CR) and prevents the individual from engaging in the compulsive behaviors that reduce negative mood. The repeated exposure without anxiety reduction causes two behavioral changes. Continued exposure to the negative mood state without escape via compulsive behaviors leads to eventual habituation to the negative feelings of anxiety, disgust, and shame elicited by the perceived flaw and the intensity of the negative feelings diminish. Breaking the negative reinforcement of compulsive and safety seeking behaviors leads to extinction of these behaviors.

This behavioral model has been used to treat many BDD patients. Below, a case study illustrates how treatment was successfully applied with one patient to explicate how the behavioral model and the treatment are intertwined.

4. Case study

Chris, a 19 year old male, presented for intensive treatment expressing excessive concerns about the appearance of his nose. Prior to age 17, Chris reports having been socially active, popular, and happy. At the age of 16, he broke his nose while playing ice hockey, after which he had cosmetic surgery to repair the damage to his nose. Since the surgery, Chris has been preoccupied with fears that his nose was changing shape and collapsing on the left side. He believed that defects in his nose were extremely offensive and visible to all. Anxiety related to his perceived flaw interfered with his interpersonal relationships, social life, and education. Chris began to drink heavily so he could tolerate discomfort in social situations.

Chris spent several hours each day engaging in mirror checking and camouflaging behaviors. He wore hats to create a shadow on his face and detract attention from his nose. On multiple occasions, Chris would apply tinted moisturizer in an attempt to correct his defect. Additionally, he would take countless photographs of his nose, until he found one that he felt was bearable. Eventually, the anxiety, disgust, and shame related to his perceived defect became unbearable, and he dropped out of school and avoided most social contact, except his parents, remaining in his home most days and nights.

4.1 Case conceptualization

4.1.1 Biological predisposition and social learning

In discussing his family history, Chris reported a strong family focus on appearance and attractiveness. He reported that his mother and sisters were highly focused looking perfectly put together, and that his mother had been diagnosed with a mild case of obsessive-compulsive disorder, supporting a possible biological predisposition in his family.

4.1.2 Early childhood reinforcement history

Chris reported that throughout his childhood, his appearance was exaggerated to the exclusion of other personality traits and behavioral accomplishments. He was positively reinforced (operant conditioning) for his good looks. As a child, he modeled for clothing catalogues and often went shopping with his mother. These appearance based activities were central to his relationship with his mother. Chris reports that prior to his emergence of BDD symptoms, he engaged in appearance related behaviors, such as styling his hair daily, as well as non-compulsive mirror checking. He was rather popular in his social group and received significant positive attention from friends and girlfriends for his appearance.

4.2 Symptom development and maintenance

4.2.1 Classical conditioning

After Chris's surgery, he began to feel differently about his appearance. The change in his appearance (broken nose), the pain and discomfort from the surgery (US) became associated with disgust and anxiety (UR). His nose then (CS) became associated with these negative mood states (CR).

4.2.2 Operant conditioning

Chris began to avoid the anxiety and disgust associated with his appearance. He engaged in various behaviors such as mirror checking, taking multiple photographs of his nose, camouflaging with hats and make-up, social avoidance, and excessive drinking. Chris's compulsions were strengthened and maintained via negative reinforcement (the avoidance of a negative outcome- anxiety, shame, social rejection, etc.).

5. Treatment

5.1 Treatment frequency

Initially treatment consisted of 3 hour sessions 5 times a week. After 6 weeks, frequency was reduced to 90 minute sessions 4-5 times a week. As Chris experienced symptom reduction, he was seen on average twice a week for 90 minutes.

5.2 Treatment content

The initial treatment sessions concentrated on gathering information about Chris' symptoms as well as providing psychoeducation about BDD. As ERP involves exposure to the most anxiety provoking situations, trust between the patient and therapist is necessary. Therefore, the initial sessions also focused on rapport building and engaging Chris in treatment. His motivation wavered as is typical of BDD individuals.

The above model stresses that BDD is maintained through both classical and operant conditioning principles such as habituation and exposure. These principles are applied in order to treat BDD and reverse pathological behavior patterns. Chris must unlearn all of his previously conditioned responses and learn new responses.

First, information was collected and used to create a hierarchy of situations that elicited negative mood states such as feelings of disgust and anxiety about his appearance in which he would normally engage in compulsions and safety behaviors to avoid these negative feelings. Chris rated the situations from lowest to highest based on how much anxiety, disgust, and distress each caused. The ERP exercises were designed to (a) help the patient habituate to his anxiety and other negative emotions in the presence of the conditioned stimuli (e.g. his nose and the chance that others may scrutinize him) and (b) extinguish his compulsive and safety seeking behaviors. To challenge his avoidance and belief that others only saw his defect, exposures were designed around anxiety-provoking situations in which Chris felt his flaw was most prominent. The ERP exercises involved extensive social interactions in which Chris was not allowed to engage in camouflaging behaviors. For example, an early exposure consisted of Chris sitting in the waiting room for treatment without a hat on. By extending his time without camouflaging, Chris habituated to his anxiety in that situation and to the accompanying negative feelings of anxiety, disgust, and shame about being seen in public. Similar exposures were conducted across various settings (e.g. while driving in the car, at a movie theatre, and in a coffee shop). He was able to extinguish the camouflage behavior and wearing his hat whenever he was in a public place. A later exposure involved approaching and engaging salespeople in a department store without camouflage. This allowed habituation to the negative emotions when in closer proximity to others and extinction of the camouflage behavior when engaged in one on one interactions. ERP exercises also involved decreasing the frequency and length of Chris's mirror checking and photographing behaviors. This was done by exposing Chris with verbal negative prompts by his appearance in the presence of a mirror without letting him look and habituating to the negative feelings the verbal prompts and his appearance elicited. Chris was taught to practice quick mirror checks even in the presence of his "defect" to extinguish obsessive time consuming mirror checking behaviors.

In addition to previously learned behaviors, Chris was provided with new conditioning experiences in which he could challenge previously learned irrational beliefs and behaviors and learn appropriate and healthy interactions. Assertiveness training was provided as part of the exposure exercises at local coffee houses and bars in order in help the patient in developing the social skills lost due to the Chris's substance use when in social situations. He learned how to approach others, initiate conversations with confidence, and maintain a conversation. Positive reinforcement provided by the therapist and conversation recipient increased Chris's confidence and decreased the previously negative emotions associated with social interactions.

During treatment, Chris's beliefs were challenged as well. For example, Chris believed that his job and relationship success were dependent on his physical attractiveness. He felt that without a perfectly straight nose he would never be able to make friends, have a girlfriend, or finish school. These thoughts were challenged by providing empirical evidence and corrective feedback. For example, Chris's irrational beliefs about the importance of appearance for success were challenged with examples of how others have succeeded without physical perfection. To empirically challenge Chris's beliefs, we gave photo's of Chris's nose (one in which he thought his nose looked "acceptable" and one in which his "deformity" was prominent) to third party individuals and had them rate the attractiveness of the photo. The rating of the attractiveness did not change from photo to photo. By combining ERP and exercises to challenge Chris's cognition distortions, he was able to decrease his BDD symptoms.

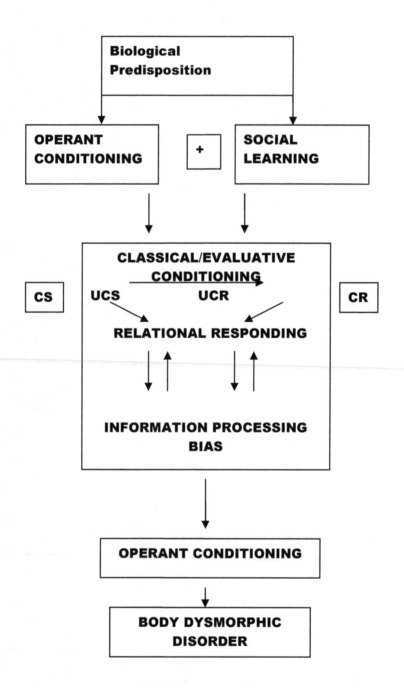

Fig. 1.

6. Conclusion

While there is no leading model of BDD formulation, the aforementioned CBT model of BDD attempts to explain the development and maintenance of BDD symptoms. The CBT model based on learning suggests that a biological predisposition along with early learning experiences via direct reinforcement and vicarious learning can lead to BDD symptoms. Additionally, relational frames may play a role in the development in BDD. It is how an individual associates events based on their learning experiences. Once BDD symptoms are developed, they are maintained via negative reinforcement. ERP coupled with cognitive therapy is an efficacious treatment approach. Repeated exposures to beliefs, behaviors, and negative emotions while preventing learned escape and avoidance behaviors can aid the BDD individual in habituation and extinction of BDD behaviors, and prepare the individual to re-learn healthy behaviors.

7. References

American Psychiatric Association. (2000). *Diagnostic and statistical manual of mental disorders* (4th ed.-Text Revision). Washington, DC: Author

American Psychiatric Association. (1987). *Diagnostic and statistical manual of mental disorders* (3rd edition). Washington, DC: Author

Bandura, A. (1977). *Social learning theory*. Prentice Hall: Englewood Cliffs, NJ.

Cash, T.F. (2002). Cognitive behavioral perspectives on body image. In T. F. Cash & T. Pruzinsky (Eds.), *Body image: A handbook of theory, research, and clinical practice* (pp. 14-38). New York: Guilford Press.

Feusner, J. D., Townsend, J., Bystritsky, A. 7 Bookheimer, S. (2007). Visual Information Processing of Faces In Body Dysmorphic Disorder. *Archives of General Psychiatry*, 64(12), 334-349.

Feusner, J. D., Yaryura-Tobia, J., & Saxena, S. (2008). The pathophysiology of body Dysmorphic disorder. *Body Image, 5*, 3-12.

Gunstad, J., & Phillips, K. A. (2003). Axis I comorbidity in body dysmorphic disorder. *Comprehensive Psychiatry, 44*, 270-276.

Hayes, S.C., Barnes-Holmes, D., & Roche, D. (Eds.). (2001). *Relational frame theory: A post-skinnerian account of human language and cognition*. New York: Plenum Press.

McKay, D. & Neziroglu, F. (2011). Body dysmorphic disorder. In B. B. Brown and M. J. Prinstein (Eds.). *Encyclopedia of adolescence, vol. 3*. (pp.85-89). San Diego: Academic Press.

Morselli, E. (1891). Sulla dismorfofobia e sulla tafefobia. *Boll Accad Med (Genova), VI*, 110-119.

Neziroglu, F., Khemlani-Patel, S., & Jacofsky, M. (2009). Body dysmorphic disorder: Symptoms, models and treatment interventions. In S. Gregoris (Ed.) *Cognitive behaviour Therapy: A guide for the practising clinician*, (pp. 94-111). London:Routledge.

Neziroglu, F., Khemlani-Patel, S., & Veale, D. (2008) Social learning theory and cognitive behavioral models of body dysmorphic disorder. *Body Image, 5*, 28-38.

Neziroglu, F., Roberts, M. and Yaryura-Tobias, J. (2004). A behavioral model for body dysmorphic disorder. *Psychiatric Annals, 34 (12)*, 915-920.

Phillips, K. A., & Menard, W. (2006). Suicidailty in body dysmorphic disorder: A preospective study. *American Journal of Psychiatry, 163*, 1280-1282.

Phillips, K. A. (1996a). *The broken mirror – Understanding and treating body dysmorphic disorder.* New York: Oxford University Press.

Osman, S., Cooper, M., Hackmann, A. & Veale, D. (2004). Spontaneously occurring images and early memories in people with body dysmorphic disorder. *Memory, 12,* 428-436.

Rabinowitz, D., Neziroglu, F., & Roberts, M. (2007) Clinical application of a behavioral model for the treatment of body dysmorphic disorder. *Cognitive and Behavioral Practice, 14,* 231-237.

Rauch, S. L., Phillips, K.A. Segal, E., Makris, E., Shin, L.M., Whalen, P. J. et al.(2003). A preliminary morphometric magnetic resonance imaging study of regional brain volumes in body dysmorphic disorder. *Psychiatry Research: Neuroimaging* 122, 13-19.

Saxena, S. & Feusner, J. D. (2006). Toward a neurobiology of body dysmorphic disorder. *Primary Psychiatry, 26(2),* 161-167.

Veale, D., Ennis, M., & Lambrou, C. (2002). Possible association of body dysmorphic disorder with an occupation or education in art and design. *American Journal of Psychiatry, 159(10),* 1788-1790.

Veale, D., & Neziroglu, F. (2010). Body Dysmorphic Disorder: A Treatment Manual, Chichester, UK: John Wiley & Sons Ltd.

Wilhelm, S., Neziroglu, F. (2002). Cognitive theory of body dysmorphic disorder. In R.O. Frost & G. Steketee (Eds.), *Cognitive approaches to obsessions and compulsions: Theory, assessment, and treatment.* (pp. 203-214). Amsterdam: Pergamon/ Elsevier Science.

Yaryura-Tobias, J.A., Neziroglu, F., Chang, R., Lee, S., Pinto, A & Donohue, L. (2002) Computerized perceptual analysis of patients with body dysmorphic disorder: A pilot study. *CNS Spectrums, 7(6),* 444-446.

Yaryura-Tobias, J.A., Neziroglu, F., & Torres-Gallegos, M. (2002). Neuroanatomical correlates and somatosensorial disturbances in body dysmorphic disorder. *CNS Spectrums, 7(6),* 432-434.

10

Internet Addiction and Its Cognitive Behavioral Therapy

Ömer Şenormancı[1], Ramazan Konkan[1] and Mehmet Zihni Sungur[2]
[1]Bakırköy Research and Training Hospital for Psychiatry, Neurology and Neurosurgery,
[2]Marmara University School of Medicine,
Turkey

1. Introduction

Internet addiction or problematic internet use is one of the newest areas of interest in psychiatry. The internet which was developed to increase communication and facilitate information exchange has grown beyond expectations making some users unable to control their internet use and thus experience problems in their functioning at work and in social and private spheres (Young 1999). The reasons for the internet becoming so widespread in such a short time have been the subject of many studies. To explain the increase in internet use for sexual pursuits, Cooper has defined a 'Triple A Engine' (Access, Affordability and Anonymity). Access is the ease of having access to the internet anywhere and anytime and finding whatever is sought in the internet where there is no refusal. Affordability is the ease of having access to the rich content of the internet especially in on-line sexuality in return for an affordable price. Anonymity is the secrecy of an individual's both real and perceived identity (Cooper 1998). These popularizing and facilitating factors may enable us to understand the increase in using the internet in all other areas.

Such a big increase in internet use resulted in problematic use and even addiction for some individuals. Problems relating to excessive and abusive use of the internet have been defined as excessive cognitive involvement associated with the use of the internet, recurring thoughts about limiting and controlling the use, inability to cease craving for access, persistence in using the internet in spite of impaired functioning at various levels, spending increasingly more time in the internet and longing and craving behaviors when there is no possibility of using it (Young 1999).

Although such abuse of the internet is not included in DSM-IV-TR, the classification system of the American Psychiatric Association, there is a tendency to call it 'internet addiction'. There are proposals to include internet addiction as a disorder in the new DSM-V to be prepared (Block 2008). Various names were given to the uncontrolled use of the internet such as 'computer addiction', 'online addiction', 'cyber addiction', 'pathological internet use', 'excessive internet use', 'internet addiction disorder', 'net addiction', 'cyberspace addiction', 'problematic internet use', 'technologic addiction', 'compulsive internet use' and 'internet behavior addiction' (Hall and Parsons 2001; Caplan 2002; Davis et al. 2002; Whang et al. 2003; Lee and Shin 2004; Hur 2006; Widyanto and Griffiths 2007).

2. Background of the definition of internet addiction

Although internet addiction is a subject attracting extensive attention, debates on its existence are still continuing (Korkeila et al. 2009). The person who defined 'internet addiction' and tried to identify the diagnosis criteria for the first time is Goldberg. To criticize the rigidity of the DSM system Goldberg jokingly adapted the substance addiction criteria in DSM-IV to uncontrolled internet use and published them in his own website. Such criteria include fantasies and dreams about internet use as well as voluntary and involuntary finger movements (Goldberg 1995). Young, on the other hand, concluded that the disorder closest to internet addiction in DSM-IV was 'pathological gambling' under the heading 'impulse control disorders' because the non-intoxicant behavioral addictions were considered as impulse control disorders in DSM-IV and specified the criteria for internet addiction on the basis of such pathological gambling criteria. Although there were 10 criteria for pathological gambling, two of them were excluded for being inadaptable to internet use and 8 criteria in total were included in the diagnosis criteria. Young found at least 5 or more answers of yes to these 8 criteria sufficient for internet addiction (Table 1) (Young 1998).

---

1. Do you feel preoccupied with the Internet (think about previous on-line activity or anticipate next on-line session)?
2. Do you feel the need to use the Internet with increasing amounts of time in order to achieve satisfaction?
3. Have you repeatedly made unsuccessful efforts to control, cut back, or stop Internet use?
4. Do you feel restless, moody, depressed, or irritable when attempting to cut down or stop Internet use?
5. Do you stay on-line longer than originally intended?
6. Have you jeopardized or risked the loss of significant relationship, job, educational or career opportunity because of the Internet?
7. Have you lied to family members, therapist, or others to conceal the extent of involvement with the Internet?
8. Do you use the Internet as a way of escaping from problems or of relieving a dysphoric mood (e.g., feelings of helplessness, guilt, anxiety, depression)?

Table 1. Young's Criteria for Internet Addiction.

Beard and Wolf stated that the first five criteria defined by Young could be met without any loss of functioning in a person and thus at least one of the last three criteria (criterion 6, 7 or 8), which are directly related to functioning, should also be met (Beard and Wolf 2001). Like Young, Beard and Wolf, Shapira and associates also considered internet addiction as a impulse control disorder and pointed out that the exclusion criteria which is excessive internet use does not occur exclusively during periods of hypomania or mania and is not better accounted for by other Axis 1 disorders should especially be taken into account among the diagnosis criteria they devised (Shapira et al. 2003). Brenner defined internet addiction by adapting DSM-IV substance addiction criteria in 32 items of right or wrong and Anderson in 7 items of right or wrong (Brenner 1997; Anderson 2001). Aboujaoude and associates combined the impulse control disorders, obsessive compulsive disorder, substance abuse and the abovementioned internet addiction criteria and developed their four-step diagnosis criteria (Aboujaoude et al. 2006).

More studies in different fields are being carried out in recent years towards understanding the etiologic roots of internet addiction. In a genetic study where internet addicts were compared to a control group to identify the biologic origin of the disorder, the group consisting of internet addicts was found to have markedly shorter alleles in their serotonin-carrying genes and higher scores of harm avoidance and depression (Lee et al. 2008). In another study of brain imaging made on internet addicts, the addicts had less concentrations of grey matter in their left anterior cingulate cortex, left posterior cingulate cortex, left insula and left lingual gyrus as compared to the control group (Zhou et al. 2009). In an electro-physiologic trial on internet addiction, the addicted group was observed to make more cognitive effort to complete their assignments and to have lower efficiency in processing information and less impulse control as compared to the control group (Dong et al. 2010). It was reported in a neuro-cognitive study of internet addiction that the findings of internet addiction did not resemble those of substance addiction or pathological gambling in spite of all those efforts to diagnose internet addiction within the DSM system (Ko et al. 2010).

3. Epidemiology

The prevalence of internet addiction was reported to be between 1.5% and 8.2% (Peterson 2009). We can give 3 examples of studies from 3 different cultures where different scales were used: The prevalence of internet addiction was found to be 1.98% in a study made in Norway on 3237 adolescents between 12 and 18 years of age who used and did not use the internet by employing Young's 'Diagnostic Questionnaire for Internet Addiction – YDQ' (Johansson and Götestam 2004). The prevalence of pathological internet use was found to be 8.1% in a study carried out in the USA on 277 collage students including six participants who had not previously used the internet by employing a 'Pathological Internet Use Scale – PIUS' (Morahan-Martin and Schumacher 2000). The prevalence of internet addiction was observed to be 17.9% in another study made in Taiwan on 4710 university freshmen who agreed to take part in the study by employing the 'Chinese Internet Addiction Scale-Revision – CIAS-R' (Tsai et al. 2009).

Considering the gender difference, clinical samplings as well as society-based and online studies revealed that internet addiction was more in men. Although studies show that internet addiction starts in late 20's and early 30's, the natural trend of internet addiction is not fully known yet (Shaw and Black 2008).

The studies made on internet addiction may have produced inconsistent results for reasons such as the scales used in such studies, scales being used failing to measure the intensity of addiction, scales not having time dimension, inclination of some individuals to minimize their problems in self-reporting scales, most of the studies tending to exaggerate the problem and failing to differentiate for what reason the internet is being used (it may be for the purpose of work or communicating with some distant associate), invalid and unreliable research methods, target population and differences in cultural and social structures (Widyanto and Griffiths 2007; Tsai et al. 2009; Huang et al. 2010).

4. Comorbidity

Block stated that in 86% of those diagnosed as having internet addiction had also another DSM-IV diagnosis and pointing out that an average of 1.5 additional diagnoses were found per person per study he said the problem became increasingly complicated in comorbid diseases (Block 2008). The studies made in this area reported that comorbid situations encountered in internet addiction included social phobia, depression, anxiety disorders, shyness, introversion, loneliness, personality disorders, substance addiction, sexual compulsivity and attention deficit and hyperactivity disorder (ADHD) (Robin-Marie Shepherd et al. 2005; Kratzer et al. 2008; Saunders et al. 2008; Ebeling-Witte et al. 2007; Yoo et al. 2004; Kraut et al. 1998; Cooper et al. 1999; Morahan-Martin and Schumacher 2000; Shapira et al. 2000). I It was reported that excessive use of technology during adolescence (as in mailing) might relate to the risk of increased smoking and use of alcohol and this risk was more especially for those children having alcohol addicted parents (Ohannessian 2009). In a study made on 1204 male and 910 female students with ages ranging from 15 to 23 (mean 16.26), it was reported that attention deficit and hyperactivity disorder (ADHD), depression, social phobia and hostility accompanied internet addiction more frequently in boys whereas ADHD and depression were seen more often together with internet addiction in girls (Yen et al. 2007).

Comorbidity of two disorders does not determine the etiologic explanation. Since there are a limited number of studies on internet abuse, it may be more meaningful to accept the coexistence of internet abuse and other psycho-pathologies without considering one as the cause or symptom of the other (Morahan-Martin 2005).

5. Materials used in diagnoses and studies

There are no diagnosis criteria for internet addiction. A large number of scales were developed and used for internet addiction in studies. Examples of such scales include Young's 'Internet Addiction Test – IAT' (Young 1998b), 'Diagnostic Questionnaire for Internet Addiction – YDQ' (Petersen et al. 2009), 'Pathological Internet Use Scale – PIUS' (Johansson and Götestam 2004), 'Chinese Internet Addiction Scale-Revision – CIAS-R' (Tsai et al. 2009) and 'Distinguishing Characteristics of Internet Addiction – DC-IA-C' (Ko et al. 2009). In a trial systematically investigating the psychometric aspects of the Internet Addiction Test – IAT, 6 factors came to the fore, which are salience, excessive use, neglecting work, anticipation, lack of control and neglecting social life. These factors were found to have good validity and internal consistency, salience being the most reliable item (Widyanto and McMurran 2004). It was demonstrated that the Internet Addiction Test – IAT was also valid in different cultures (Korkeila et al. 2009).

6. Subtypes of internet addiction

Some investigators report that uncontrolled internet users are not really internet addicts but addicts of material such as gambling, chatting, shopping and gaming they can get from the internet. Therefore, it is important to differentiate the real internet addicts from those who satisfy their other addictions through the internet (Griffiths 2000; Li and Chung 2006).

As a result of her study on 35 people, Young divided internet addiction into 5 subtypes. These are cybersex addiction, cyber-relationship addiction, net compulsions, information overload and computer addiction. Cybersex addiction typically involves watching, downloading, online porno exchange or role plays of sexual fantasies in chat rooms. Cyber-relationship addiction may relate to establishment of excessive online relationships or virtual sex. Online relationships come to get more important than those in real life. Net Compulsions involves a broad category of subtype behaviors including online gambling, shopping and trading. It may result in large amounts of financial loss. Information Overload relates to spending of excessive time for searching for, gathering and organizing information (compulsive web surfing or database search). Computer addiction is addiction to the games loaded in the computer (e.g. doom, myst or solitaire). Employees tend to spend their working hours on these games rather than on their work (Young et al. 1999; Shaw and Black 2008).

Like Young, Davis also preferred the term pathological internet use to describe uncontrolled/excessive internet use. Davis divided the internet into two as 'specific' and 'generalized' according to the purpose of using it (Table 2) (Davis 2001).

Specific	Generalized
• They are addicted to a specific function of the internet among its many functions • It involves online sexual material/services, online auction services, online stock trading, and online gambling • It is assumed to be the result of a previously developed psycho-pathology • It continues in the absence of the internet because it is content-specific • Internet use for addicts is nothing but an expression of devotion to various stimuli	• It involves general and multi-purpose use of the internet • It relates to the social aspect of the internet • It emerges particularly as a result of a lack of social support from the family or friends, or a social isolation • It involves pastime such as online chats and e-mails with no definite purpose • The social contact and support occurring online result in an intense desire to remain in such artificial social life • Those with intense internet addiction use the internet to postpone their responsibilities • There is no way for them to express their anxiety, the internet is the connection of the individual with the outer world

Table 2. Subtypes of Internet Addiction.

7. Models proposed for etiology of internet addiction

In order to develop effective methods in treating internet addiction, the underlying mechanisms should be understood very well. One of the most comprehensive studies made towards this end is the cognitive behavioral model designed by Davis. This model places maladaptive cognitions in the center of pathologic internet use. While the scope of the behavior and the negative effects of this behavior on daily life were emphasized in the previous internet addiction studies, this model also focuses on maladaptive cognitions (Davis 2001).

The cognitive behavioral model of internet addiction defines the healthy use of the internet as a manner of using the internet for a clear purpose for a period of time that can be considered reasonable under the conditions specific to the user and in recognition of the differences between the real communication and the communication through the internet without assuming a different personality (Davis 2001).

Some basic concepts need to be understood before explaining the cognitive theory of pathological internet use (PIU). In his cognitive behavioral theory, Davis initially used some basic concepts described by Abramson and associates to define the factors contributing to PIU. The factors inducing the behavior were classified as 'necessary', 'sufficient' and 'contributory'. A necessary factor is the etiologic factor that should exist for the symptoms to appear. A necessary etiologic factor is necessary in the context of development of a set of symptoms, but existence of such etiologic factors may not necessarily produce the symptoms. In other words, these factors are necessary but not sufficient in occurrence of pathology. Sufficient factors are etiologic causes, the existence of which guarantees occurrence of the symptoms. A contributory factor is an etiologic cause, the existence of which greatly increases occurrence of various symptoms, but is not necessary or sufficient for occurrence of pathology. Abramson et al. divided the causes into two as proximal and distal depending on the closeness of the pathological behavior to the segment where it occurred along the etiologic chain that results in a set of symptoms. They stated that in the etiologic chain that results in a set of symptoms, some causes were lie towards the end of the chain (proximal) and others close to beginning of the chain but at a point distant from the symptom (distal). If we were to exemplify these concepts using occurrence of anxiety symptoms such as increase in the heart rate, sweating and dryness in the mouth, we can give stress, danger or other fear-inducing situations as examples of proximal causes. Examples of distal causes may include sleeplessness, cardiac arrhythmia and paranoia caused by drugs. Thus, sleeplessness can be considered as a contributory cause distant to the anxiety symptoms for both being insufficient to be a cause of the symptoms and not being closely attributable to the anxiety symptoms under the name of 'etiology'. By contrast, a life-threatening situation may be a proximal and sufficient cause of the anxiety symptoms, because it is sufficient to create anxiety by itself. In other words, it is closely associated with the physical symptoms of an autonomic stimulation and thus with anxiety (Davis 2001).

7.1 Distal causes

Distal contributory causes of PIU have been explained within the framework of a diathesis-stress model. The cognitive-behavioral model of PIU (Figure 1) asserts that psychopathology is a distal necessary cause of PIU symptoms, meaning that psychopathology is 'definitely necessary' for PIU symptoms. It should be noted that the underlying psychopathology alone does not result in PIU symptoms, but may be the necessary cause in etiology. The stressor in this model is the introduction of the internet or of some new technologies in the internet. Such first encounter may be the discovery of pornography in the internet, a first-time e-chat, first-time shopping in the internet or online trading in the stock exchange. Exposure to such technologies is a distal necessary cause for PIU symptoms. The key incidence in experiencing the internet and the related technologies is the positive experience attained by the individual from that event. In other words, if the response to experiencing a new function of the internet is positive, it reinforces the continuity of activity. This operant conditioning continues until the person finds new technologies to have similar physiologic response. During the normal course of this conditioning, another conditioning towards associated stimuli may also occur. According to the principles of operant conditioning, any stimulus that is associated with the original conditioning stimulus may produce the same reactions through a secondary reinforcement. For example, stimuli such as the sound of a computer connecting to the internet, the sensation of touching when typing on the keyboard and the scent of the room may produce the same satisfaction through conditioned responses. The secondary reinforcements are the factors that help develop and sustain situational cues which reinforce occurrence of PIU symptoms (Davis 2001).

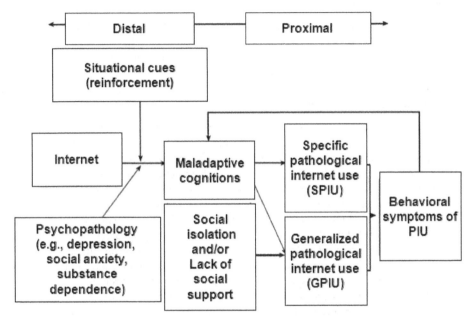

*Davis RA. 'A cognitive-behavioral model of pathological Internet use.' Comput Hum Behav 2001; 17:187-195.

Fig. 1. The cognitive behavior model used by Davis to describe Internet addiction*.

7.2 Proximal causes

The most fundamental component of PIU are the non-functional ruminative cognitions of self. Ruminations relate to a person's thinking in a way to repeat the problems in internet use rather than directing his/her attention to the other events in his/her life. A person's constant efforts to understand why he/she uses the internet in an excessive way involve thoughts and behaviors such as reading about PIU or talking to friends about excessive use of the internet. It delays the interpersonal problem solving behavior and causes a stronger recall of the person's internet-related memories by preventing effective behavior such as taking action for implementing a plan. In this way, it causes the vicious circle within PIU to prevail in an aggravated way. These individuals have a negative point of view about themselves and use the internet to get positive responses from other people without taking a risk. They usually have 'excessive generalizations' and 'all-or-nothing' type of thought patterns about themselves and the outer world. They tend to have automatic thoughts about themselves such as 'I am good only at internet', 'I am useless when I am not in the internet, but I am an important person in the internet' and 'I am a failure when I am not in the internet' and about the outer world such as 'The only place where I am respected is the internet', 'Nobody likes me when I am not in the internet', 'The internet is my only friend' and 'People treat me badly outside the internet environment' (Davis 2001). The addicts are more inclined towards catastrophizing and anxiety than other people. Young argued that the avoidance of real and perceived consequences of catastrophizing also contributes to compulsive use of the internet (Young 2007).

Based on the extensive use of PIU concept proposed by the Davis model, Caplan has made studies on university students using the 'Generalized Problematic Internet Use Scale' he developed. The study results revealed that people with low self-esteem were alone, they preferred to establish social relationships through the internet instead of face-to-face communication and this played a role in the etiology, development and outcomes of extensive pathologic internet use (Caplan 2002).

Douglas and associates have reviewed the articles published between 1996 and 2006 by way of meta-synthesis and proposed a conceptual internet addiction model. According to this model, excessive internet use is determined by mostly internal requirements and the individual's motivation (push factors such as ability to conceal identity, distress relieving and relaxing effect and meeting social needs). However, personal inclination is also important (antecedents such as being in environments allowing internet use like student hostels, internet use for many years and feeling of being misunderstood by others, and addict profiles such as refusal of excessive internet use as being a problem and having very little or no social life and/or self-confidence). The model mentions that the perceived attractive aspects of the environment (pull factors such as online gambling, access to addictive applications like games and chat, easy access to the internet and to information through the internet, ease of social interaction and idea exchange and easier communication through the internet as compared to other media) and the push factors ease the relationship between the excessive use of internet and the severity of the negative effects. Besides academic, social, economic and occupational effects and physical effects such as changes in sleeping patterns, the negative effects of internet addiction may also involve deviant behaviors (online porno, online stock exchange, virtual sex instead of normal relations and social activities for those with extreme shyness). The individual's awareness of the problem of internet addiction may facilitate use of control strategies to prevent the addiction. Some individuals are more likely to adopt behaviors deviated from the normal than others, thus a direct connection was proposed between the antecedents and the behaviors deviated from the normal (Figure 2) (Douglas et al. 2008).

Spada and associates investigated meta-cognitions as the mediator of the relationship between PIU and negative feelings (boredom, depression, anxiety) in university students using the internet. As a result, a positive and significant relationship was found between problematic internet use and the entire five dimensions of the Meta-cognitions Questionnaire-MCQ used in the trial, namely 'positive beliefs', 'cognitive confidence', 'uncontrollability and danger', 'cognitive awareness' and 'need of control' and the negative feelings. These results support the assumption that the relationship between PIU and negative feelings is entirely mediated by meta-cognitions (Spada et al. 2008; Wells and Cartwright-Hatton 2004).

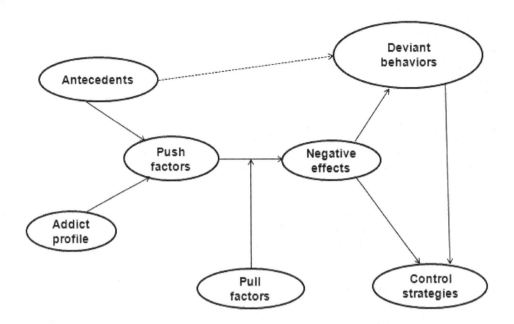

*Douglas A, Mills J, Niang M, Stepchenkova S, Byun S, Ruffini C, et al., 'Internet addiction: Meta-synthesis of qualitative research for the decade 1996-2006.' Comput Human Behav 2008; 24:3027-3044.

Fig. 2. The conceptual Internet addiction model*.

8. Treatment

Since internet addiction is a relatively new concept, there are a limited number of generally accepted and empirical treatment methods for it. The methods proposed for treatment of internet addiction consist of primarily psychotherapy and some pharmacologic interventions.

Although the underlying basic psychopathology may produce internet addiction symptoms according to the cognitive behavioral model of internet addiction, internet addiction symptoms are specific to internet addiction and basic psychopathology and internet addiction should be investigated and targeted separately (Davis 2001). Young, on the other hand, argued that some people are in depression or in depressive episode of a bipolar disorder and if the cognitions that result in addicted internet use can be detected in such people, these cases should be treated using the basic psychopathology and it should be monitored whether or not the internet use has improved after that therapy (Young 1999).

The efforts to treat internet addiction through pharmacologic therapy are limited to a few trials made in recent years. In a trial investigating the efficacy of escitalopram on internet addiction, all of the 19 participants were administered escitalopram in the first 10-week open-label phase of the trial and then they were given escitalopram and placebo in a random and double-blind way for 9 weeks during the cut-off phase. The entire group was found to have benefited from the medication treatment at the first stage, but there was no significant difference between the groups taking placebo and escitalopram at the cut-off phase (Dell'Osso et al. 2008). After over a 3-year monitoring, a serious recovery was achieved by administering naltrexone, which is an opiate antagonist inhibiting dopamine release increasing effects of opiates, to an internet sex addict who had been euphorically compulsive due to the role of the center of reward and dopamine in the addiction and whose functioning had been adversely affected (Bostwick and Bucci 2008). Craving for playing games in the internet, total gaming time and cue induced brain activity in dorsolateral prefrontal cortex decreased in 11 online gaming addicts who were administered medication therapy with Bupropion SR for 6 weeks. It was pointed out that Bupropion, which is a dopamine and norepinephrine reuptake inhibitor, was able to achieve these changes in a similar manner as in individuals with substance abuse or addiction (Han et al. 2010). In a 12-week double-blind trial involving an 8-week active treatment phase and a following 4-week post-treatment monitoring period, the effects of Bupropion and placebo were compared in 50 males with comorbid depression and online gaming addiction after administering randomized Bupropion + training to use internet or placebo + training to use internet to the participants. It was found in the trial that depression scores dropped during the active treatment, playing online games decreased and this improvement continued during the 4-week post-treatment follow-up period (Han and Renshaw 2011). Although pharmacologic studies on internet addiction are limited in number, it can be stated according to the available data that a distinct benefit from medication can be in the specific group, but psychotherapeutic interventions should be considered first in the generalized usage which relates to the social aspect of the internet.

Multi-modality therapy applications have usually been used in psychotherapy of internet addiction. The most important study that provides an idea on the effectiveness of a cognitive behavioral therapy on internet addiction and its prognosis is the study of Young where 114 internet addicts were administered only a cognitive behavioral therapy. In that study, patient motivation, online time management, improvement in social relationships, improvement in sexual functioning, ability to engage in activities outside the internet, and ability to avoid problematic applications were assessed in the 3rd, 8th and 12th sessions and in the 6th month. Clinical recovery started in most of the cases from the third session onwards and an apparent clinical improvement was achieved at the end of the 8th session. The subjects maintained their improvements during the 6-month follow-up period. The most effective improvement was in online time management in the early periods of the therapy. Social problems such as revival of non-internet relationships and engagement in non-internet activities were solved in the later periods of the therapy, generally durign the 12th session. Success was the least in non-internet sexual functioning. Many patients could keep away from sexual chats and online pornography, but they reported problems in their matrimonial relationships. During the 6-month follow-up period, 5 patients got divorced for not being able to revive a satisfactory sexual relation with their partners (Young 2007).

In a 16-week study involving a cognitive behavioral group therapy, readiness-to-change, motivational interviewing and cognitive behavioral therapy interventions were used on 35 males who used the internet for sexual pursuits. Although improvements were observed in the quality of life and depression scores, a significant improvement was not seen in internet usage. In this study the addicts were also divided into 3 categories, namely 'anxiety', 'attention deficit hyperactivity' and 'mood' to investigate the effect of comorbidity on the results of the treatment and the best results were obtained in the 'anxiety' group, whereas the 'mood' group gave relative response and the 'attention deficit hyperactivity' group did not give a distinct response (Orzack et al. 2006).

In a literature-based study conducted in China on 59 adolescents employing an 'indigenous multi-level counseling program' which involved the intervention techniques and strategies in the fields of substance abuse, family counseling and peer support groups, the problem of internet addiction was reduced after joining the program and there were positive changes in the perceived parenting of the users. A subjective assessment showed that the participants found the program useful (Shek et al. 2009).

Reality therapy encourages the clients to discover their behaviors and assess how effectively they achieve their wishes. The following questions are asked to the clients: What are you doing right now? What did you really do last month and last week? What holds you back from doing what you want? What will you do tomorrow or in the future? Kim made a study on 13 undergraduates and a 12-person control group using a group reality therapy of two sessions a week lasting 5 weeks. The control group did not receive any treatment in the study and the level of internet addiction markedly decreased in the group treated and their self-esteem increased significantly as compared to the control group (Kim 2008).

Two randomized groups were included in a study investigating the effectiveness of a cognitive behavioral group therapy in internet addiction; one of the groups had 32 subjects aged between 12 and 17 who had active treatment and the other group consisted of 24 individuals who did not have any treatment. The participants were assessed at the baseline, immediately after the school-based group CBT of 8 sessions and in the 6th month. Although internet use decreased in both groups, the multimedia school-based group had apparent improvements in time management skills as well as in emotional, cognitive and behavioral symptoms after the CBT (Du et al. 2010).

The Acceptance and Commitment Therapy (ACT) is another therapy emerged within the framework of cognitive behavioral therapy. It targets internal experiences (thoughts, emotions and bodily sensations), uses behavior changing strategies and focuses on the current problems. 6 adult men with problematic internet pornography viewing were assessed before an ACT of 8 sessions each lasting 1.5 hours and in weekly and quarterly monitoring after the therapy. The result was a marked decrease in viewing that continued during the follow-up period. Psychological flexibility measurements showed a large decline whereas thought-action fusion and thought-control measurements had a minor decline. Although the study had limitations, it was the first ACT interference that was tested for internet pornography viewing adhering to the treatment template proposed by Hayes and associates.

Although multi-modality therapy interventions produce positive results in internet addiction, it is difficult to distinguish in these studies which therapy is more effective and which is less effective.

The cognitive behavioral therapy approach, which was derived from the therapies applied to alcohol addiction and substance abuse, seems to be an effective method in treating internet addiction even though it has no empirical evidences (Young 2007).

Many close associates of patients with internet addiction seek help to find ways of treating the addiction and consult to various institutions in despair. Surprisingly, many internet addicts are not in pursue of a treatment in spite of their impaired family, work and social lives and show little awareness of their problems. As supported by study results (Orzack et al. 2006; Shek et al. 2009) along with our clinical observations, the first stage in treating internet addiction can be the use of motivational interview techniques.

Motivational interviewing is a directive and client oriented approach that is used to help discover the ambivalence of behaviors and analyze them and finally achieve changing of the behavior. Motivational interviewing is not a therapy, but an interviewing technique where a set of strategies are used to enable initiation of further therapeutic interventions (Miller and Rollnick 2002). While some patients seek treatment themselves, others may have been 'compelled to come in' by their relatives. Treating internet addiction requires a change. Different approaches should be employed according to the stage in which the individual is in the process of changing. The trans-theoretic model of behavior introduced by Prochaska and DiClemente (Figure 3), which involves the stages of pre-contemplation, contemplation, decision, action, maintenance and relapse, may help view individuals at different stages and make interventions according to those stages. Since an individual is not aware of the existence of a problem at the pre-contemplation stage, he/she may not even attempt to defend him/herself; at this stage, the therapist should strive to deal with the denial and to move on to the next stage. Information is given at this stage about healthy internet use to create a possibility of change. The advantages (Pros) and disadvantages (Cons) of computer use may be evaluated. At contemplation phase, the client agrees to change, but does not have enough desire for changing. The patient has ambivalence and the motivational interviewing techniques are useful at this stage (Christensen et al. 2001, Miller and Rollnick 2002).

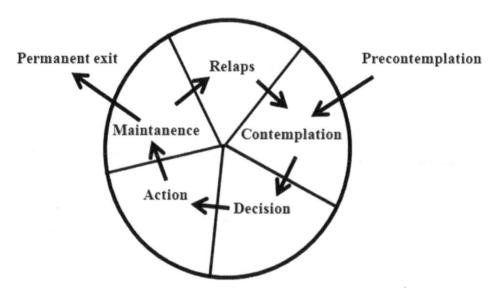

Fig. 3. Transtheoretical model of change.

It is helpful to know how the individual perceive 'importance' and 'confidence' in understanding his/her ambivalence. We can evaluate these dimensions using an importance and confidence scale with a rating from zero to ten.

How important would you say is for you to regulate your computer usage habits on a scale rated from 0 to 10 where 0 is not important at all and 10 is very important?

$$0 \quad 1 \quad 2 \quad 3 \quad 4 \quad 5 \quad 6 \quad 7 \quad 8 \quad 9 \quad 10$$

Not at all   **Extremely**
important/confident   **important/confident**

And if you decided to regulate your computer usage habits, how self-confident would you say you would be to do this on the same scale rated from 0 to 10 where 0 is I am not confident at all and 10 is I am very confident?

Although it is also possible not to show the patient a scale and explain the situation verbally, it may be more useful to discuss the issue by showing a scale or by making drawings in front of the patient. It is the best to accept ambiguity if the patient's answers add up to a very low figure. In such a situation, it may be appropriate to give information about the issue in a passive way. If the person did not give a very low figure, then he/she is asked why he/she did not give a lower figure. The answers help assess the condition in which the person is (I did not say 1 because I can succeed if I continue to …; I did not say 1 because I cannot continue like this). What will result in a higher rating is found in a reverse way (What can raise you from 4 to 7? Why did you say 4 and not 7?). It is notable that this importance and confidence application also reveals the treatment target (Miller and Rollnick 2002; Rollnick et al. 1999).

Some internet addicts may develop physical symptoms such as back stain, eye stain, impairment in sleeping pattern, carpal tunnel syndrome and weight gain associated with inactivity (Young 1998). Such physical symptoms may be used as an excuse to design collective treatment targets in individuals who deny internet addiction. For example, an adult who had basketball as his hobby and who met the internet addiction criteria could not play basketball because his index finger did not heal due to typing on the keyboard. The treatment target for this patient was set out as 'correction of his computer usage habits to the extent his broken index finger is healed and he is able to play basketball again'.

Another difference of internet addiction from substance/alcohol abuse, addiction or pathologic gambling is that the relatives of patients also lack awareness like in the pre-contemplation and contemplation phases. If a risk of substance abuse or gambling is acknowledged by the families, the parents/spouse take an alert position. They try to prevent starting doing these or if already started stopping them at an early stage. We often hear from some patients who resort to personal therapy: 'My spouse changed a lot in the last 2 years, he/she does not look at my and my child's face', 'I cannot know my child anymore, his/her lessons went upside down in the last 3 months'. The internet, which is considered to be a must in modern life, may not be recognized as a problem initially by the relatives of the addicts as lack of it is not even imagined. When the history of such individuals is questioned, it can be realized that the changes in their relatives has started after uncontrolled use of the internet. In such situations, it will be necessary to inform the family about the healthy use of internet and to encourage the internet addicts to participate in the treatment together with the family.

Since computers have important functions in daily life, treatment models that require complete avoidance of the internet are not practical. Unlike other addictions, the therapy here should involve goal-oriented techniques that encourage orderly and controlled internet use and alternative activities that keep one away from the internet (Young 2007; Young 2004). In the CBT (cognitive behavioral therapy) developed by Young, the cognitive behavioral therapy of internet addiction is limited by time as in other cognitive behavioral therapies and it usually lasts three months or 12 sessions (Young 2007). It may be advisable to make behavioral interventions during the early stages of a CBT of internet addiction.

During the therapy, a behavioral analysis is made and the case is formulated. As in other addiction types, internet use behavior is fully defined with all its aspects bearing in mind the possibility of the individual's hiding and reducing his/her complaints (especially in online sex users). In order to collect information about the internet use habits of the individual, the clinician seeks answers to the following questions: "On what days do you typically get connected to the internet? What time of the day do you usually sign in to the internet? How long do you usually stay connected in a typical login? Where do you usually use the computer?". Besides these, it should also be investigated whether the users are dependent on a specific function of the internet, because constant and frequent use of a particular function may trigger internet addiction and it can also serve as an indication for the interventions (Is it a specific internet addiction or a general one?) we intend to make during the therapy. To do this, the answers to the following questions are evaluated: "What functions of the internet are you using? How many hours on average do you allocate for each function in a week? Can you list the functions you use from the most important one to the least important one? What aspect of each function do you like the most?" (Young 1999) Other useful questions include "What do you think your problem exactly is, how do you interpret it? What are the effects of internet addiction on your living environments? What will you do that you cannot do now when you solve your internet addiction problem? (reasons directing the individual to treatment and treatment targets) Why did you come for treatment at this moment? (at his/her own will, directed by his/her relatives, changed social roles, coincidence) How long can you keep away from getting connected to the internet when you feel the desire/urge to get connected to it? (how long he/she can tolerate boredom) How did your internet addiction problem start and continue? (may have started after a loss) What are the factors affecting the continuity of your internet addiction? (alcohol, substance use, presence of others)

Behavioral interventions take precedence in the cognitive behavioral therapy of internet addiction. Simple but effective behavioral techniques are used in internet addiction on the basis of the experiences of therapists applying internet addiction therapies in private centers and the studies made on other addictions. When trying to regulate uncontrolled internet use, patients should be informed that they will experience hardship at the beginning. This is normal and should be expected. These people have had great pleasure from the internet for a long time and they will crave to get connected to the internet more frequently after the deprivation they experienced. If the time span in which a person who decided to regulate his/her internet use will be connected to the internet is left uncertain, most of the attempts to limit internet use will fail. In order to prevent relapse, the patient should be administered a reasonably structured program for 'setting goals'. The new program to be devised should be frequent but short in time to reduce craving and withdrawal. For example, a 40-hour weekly use is first reduced to 20 hours. This 20-hour period may be arranged by dividing it into specific periods of time such as between 20:00 and 22:00 hours during the week and between 13:00 and 18:00 hours at weekend. A 10-hour program can be employed between 20:00 and 23:00 hours two nights during the week and between 8:30 and 12:30 am on Sunday. A logical arrangement will make the patient feel that he/she has the control over the internet not vice versa (Young 1999).

Internet use may be regulated by 'practicing the opposite' to help the individual break through the daily routine and abandon his/her virtual habit. If the person enters the internet first thing in the morning, the clinician may propose that he/she takes a shower first; if he/she enters the internet immediately after he/she comes home in the evening, sporting after work and waiting until dinner or evening news may be proposed; if he/she uses it during the week, weekend may be proposed and vice versa; if he/she uses it without a break, having a break in 30-minute intervals may be proposed; if he/she enters the internet at a certain point of the apartment, changing the place of the computer may be proposed. To interfere with internet use, 'external stoppers' such as a thing the individual has to do at that moment or a place he/she has to go may be used. For example, if the person is supposed to leave home at 7:30, entering the internet at 6:30 is proposed. In this way, he/she will have only an hour before logging out. Setting an alarm clock near the computer may be proposed against the risk of the person's negligence of natural alerts. Patients tend to exaggerate problems they experience and overlook the ways of solving them due to their thinking disorders. 'Reminder Cards' may be used to help the patient achieve his/her target of reducing internet use. The patient sincerely writes down 5 basic problems arising from internet use and 5 basic benefits he/she will have by leaving internet use in a detailed way. They look at these cards which they may be carrying in their pockets, wallets or purses to remind themselves what they wish to avoid and what they wish to do for themselves at the point of decision making when they are attracted to internet use rather than doing something more productive and healthy (Young 1999). In order to regulate their own internet use, patients may use the filtering programs that are used by parents to protect their children from having access to sexual content of the internet or by employers to increase efficiency at workplaces. A filtering program can be arranged to automatically shut itself down when the person attempts to have access to applications such as porno sites, online chat and gaming sites. Most of the internet addicts call this experience as a 'cold shower' (Young 2004). If the patient is a specific internet addict and his/her internet use cannot be regulated, he/she is made to keep away from the specific functions of the internet he/she is addicted to. The patient should stop all his/her activities related to that function. However, the patient may use other internet functions he/she uses functionally. Abstinence is employed for those patients who have a history of addiction such as alcohol or substance use and who replaced their addictions with the internet as a physically 'safe addiction' (Young 1999). Another important point to remember when making behavioral arrangements is to replace the internet with new activities even if they may not be equally pleasurable when restricting internet use which is almost the most pleasurable thing in life for the patient at that moment. If the therapist assumes the role of a technician who applies certain behavioral techniques, the patient may show symptoms similar to grief reactions and even have a depression attack in later periods even if his/her internet use is decreased. To avoid this, the strong sides of the patient should be identified during the formulation. For example, a patient who was identified to have strong social traits and to enjoy being charitable may be proposed to assume an active role in charity associations by making use of this strong trait. It should be remembered as a general rule that reinforcing weak traits alone creates a patient population having uniform standards and resembling each other.

Behavioral exercises, behavior rehearsals, couching, desensitization, relaxation techniques, self-management and attaining new social skills are the major techniques used in internet addiction therapy (Young 2007).

During further sessions, more importance is attached to cognitive presuppositions and errors (Young 2007). The person is kept away from internet to test his/her negative and non-functional thoughts coming to mind due to not being in the internet. His/her feelings before and after accessing the internet are noted. He/she is made to come across with the internet many times during this process to observe his/her cognitive reactions. His/her automatic thoughts, changes in his/her feelings and the progress in the therapy are recorded in daily observation tables (Davis 2001). Another error often made when making cognitive exercises with patients is the set of homework assigned to the patient before he/she understands the rationale behind such homework in order to have a fast improvement or treatment. Behavioral interventions have an important role in the early sessions of cognitive behavioral therapy of internet addiction. In that period, some patients are given exercises only to identify and define their emotions and then the feelings they had before and after they enter the internet, then they are made to recognize the changes in their emotions and then comes the stage of cognitive challenging which is our main goal. All of these stages are very valuable and enhance our understanding of stimulus-thought-emotion-behavior cycle and help us learn the method enabling us to interfere with this vicious cycle.

Personal therapy is not very effective in online sex addicts in regulating their sexual functioning outside the internet or rearranging the partner relationship after internet infidelity. Similar to the findings of Young in her study of cognitive behavioral therapy in internet addiction where the success was the least in non-internet sexual functioning, the patients had problems in their marriages and some got even divorced, it was found in another study that almost half of the couples got divorced and the other half lost confidence in their relationships (Young 2007; Whitty and Carr 2005). Establishing a cause and effect relationship between partnership problems and uncontrolled internet use is difficult and having a definite judgment about the cause and the effect may produce unfavorable results in the partner relationship and individually in the patient's health. Reasons such as soothing of a person involved in a problematic relationship by telling the problems arising between the couple to the third parties through the internet, ease of expressing the negative feelings about a partner and the person being validated as a response, and monotony of the sexual life between couples may urge individuals to seek sex or infidelity in the internet (Young et al. 1999; Mileham 2007); sex or infidelity in the internet may also be seen as a result of internet addiction. In conclusion, therapies conducted by clinicians specialized in couple therapy and sexual therapy with the participation of the partner may be more useful in regulating sexual functioning of internet addicts outside the internet or regulating the couple relationship after an internet infidelity.

As in all addictions, the phases of maintenance and relapse are critical also in internet addiction. It may be useful if towards the end of a therapy the patient makes a record of the techniques that have been most beneficial for him/her during the cognitive behavioral therapy sessions and prepares his/her reminder cards and use them in future when he/she has the desire of using the internet. If small deviations occur in the newly formed internet routine, patient's relatives should be tolerant and constantly give positive feedback to the smallest effort and success of the patient towards the future. Although it may be difficult for the patient's relatives to control themselves, it is risky in terms of relapse to say things such as 'all the family suffered from your internet addiction' which reminds the patient only of his/her past bad experiences or to blame him/her for his/her past behavior while trying to give positive messages by saying for example 'it is wonderful that you are not an internet addict like you used to be, why hadn't you done it before if you were able to control your internet use?'.

The 12-step support groups give an opportunity to minimize the risk of relapse. Support groups help internet addicts strengthen their social support systems, improve their relationships outside the internet and cope with the attraction of the internet in the course of recovery (Young 2004).

9. References

Aboujaoude E, Koran LM, Gamel N, Large MD, Serpe RT. Potential markers for problematic Internet use: a telephone survey of 2513 adults. CNS Spectr 2006; 11:750-755.

Anderson KJ. Internet use among college students: an exploratory study. J Am Coll Health 2001; 50:21-26.

Beard KW, Wolf EM. Modification in the proposed diagnostic criteria for internet addiction. Cyberpsychol Behav 2001; 4:377-383.

Block JJ. Issues for DSM-V: Internet addiction. Am J Psychiatry 2008; 165:306-307.

Bostwick JM, Bucci JA: Internet sex addiction treated with naltrexone. Mayo Clin Proc 2008; 83:226-230.

Brenner V. Psychology of computer use: XLVII. Parameters of Internet use, abuse and addiction: the first 90 days of the Internet Usage Survey. Psychol Rep. 1997; 80:879-882.

Caplan SE. Problematic internet use and psychosocial well-being: development of a theory based cognitivebehavioral measurement instrument. Comput Human Behav 2002; 18:553-575.

Christensen MH, Orzack MH, Babington LM, Patsoaughter CA Computer addiction. When monitor becomes control center. J Psychosoc Nurs Ment Health Serv. 2001; 39:40-47.

Cooper A, Putnam D, Planchon L, Boies S. Online sexual compulsivity: Getting tangled in the Net. Sexual Addiction and Compulsivity 1999; 6:79-104.

Cooper A. Sexuality and the Internet: Surfing into the New Millennium. Cyberpsychol Behav 1998; 1:187-193.

Davis RA. A cognitive-behavioral model of pathological Internet use. Comput Hum Behav 2001; 17:187-195.

Davis RA, Flett GL, Besser A. Validation of a new scale for measuring problematic internet use: implications for pre-employment screening. Cyberpsychology Behavior. 2002; 5: 331-345.

Dell'Osso B, Hadley SJ, Allen A, Baker B, Chaplin WF, Hollander E. Escitalopram in the treatment of impulsive-compulsive internet usage disorder: an open-label trial followed by a double-blind discontinuation phase. J Clin Psychiatry 2008; 69:452-456.

Dong G, Lu Q, Zhou H, Zhao X. Impulse inhibition in people with Internet addiction disorder: Electrophysiological evidence from a Go/NoGo study. Neurosci Lett 2010; 485:138-142.

Douglas A, Mills J, Niang M, Stepchenkova S, Byun S, Ruffini C, et al. Internet addiction: Meta-synthesis of qualitative research for the decade 1996-2006. Comput Human Behav 2008; 24:3027-3044.

Du YS, Jiang W, Vance A. Longer term effect of randomized, controlled group cognitive behavioural therapy for Internet addiction in adolescent students in Shanghai. Aust N Z J Psychiatry 2010; 44:129-134.

Ebeling-Witte S, Frank ML, Lester D. Shyness, Internet use, and personality. Cyberpsychol Behav 2007; 10:713-716.

Goldberg I. İnternet addiction disorder. 1995. Available at http://www.psycom.net/iasg.html (03.06.2009)

Griffiths M. Internet addiction: Time to be taken seriously? Addict Res Theory 2000; 8: 413-418.

Hall AS, Parsons J. Internet addiction: College student case study using best practices in cognitive behavior therapy. J Mental Health Couns 2001; 23:312-327.

Han DH, Hwang JW, Renshaw PF. Bupropion sustained release treatment decreases craving for video games and cue-induced brain activity in patients with Internet video game addiction. Exp Clin Psychopharmacol 2010; 18:297-304.

Han DH, Renshaw PF. Bupropion in the treatment of problematic online game play in patients with major depressive disorder. J Psychopharmacol Epub 2011.

Huang XQ, Li MC, Tao R. Treatment of internet addiction. Curr Psychiatry Rep 2010; 12:462-470.

Hur M. Demographic, habitual, and socioeconomic determinants of Internet addiction disorder: An empirical study of Korean teenagers. Cyberpsychol Behav 2006; 9:514-525.

Johansson A, Götestam KG. Internet addiction: characteristics of a questionnaire and prevalence in Norwegian young (12-18 years). Scand J Psychol 2004; 45:223- 229.

Kim JU. The effect of a R/T group counseling program on the Internet addiction level and self-esteem of Internet addiction university students. Int J Real Ther 2008; 27:4-12.

Ko CH, Hsiao S, Liu GC, Yen JY, Yang MJ, Yen CF. The characteristics of decision making, potential to take risks, and personality of college students with Internet addiction. Psychiatr Res 2010; 175:121-125.

Ko CH, Yen JY, Chen SH, Yang MJ, Lin HC, Yen CF. Proposed diagnostic criteria and the screening and diagnosing tool of Internet addiction in college students. Compr Psychiatry. 2009; 50:378-84. Epub 2009.

Korkeila J, Kaarlas S, Jaaskelainen M, Vahlberg T, Taiminen T. Attached to the web-harmful use of the Internet and its correlates. Eur Psychiatry 2009; 25:236-241.

Kratzer S, Hegerl U. Is "Internet Addiction" a disorder of its own?--a study on subjects with excessive internet use. Psychiatr Prax 2008; 35:80-83.

Kraut R, Patterson M, Lundmark V, Kiesler S, Mukopadhyay T, Scherlis W. Internet paradox. A social technology that reduces social involvement and psychological well-being? Am Psychol 1998; 53:1017-1031.

Lee O, Shin M. Addictive consumption of avatars in cyberspace. Cyberpsychol Behav 2004; 7:417-420.

Lee YS, Han DH, Yang KC, Daniels MA, Na C, Kee BS, Renshaw PF. Depression like characteristics of 5HTTLPR polymorphism and temperament in excessive internet users. J Affect Disord 2008; 109:165-169. Epub 2007.

Li SM, Chung TM. Internet function and Internet addictive behavior. Comput Human Behav 2006; 22: 1067-1071.

Mileham B. Online infidelity in internet chat rooms: An ethnographic exploration. Comput Human Behavior 2007; 23:11-31.

Miller WR, Rollnick S. Motivational interviewing: Preparing people for change. New York: Guilford Press, 2002.

Morahan-Martin J. Internet abuse: Addiction? Disorder? Symptom? Alternative explanations? Soc Sci Comput Rev 2005; 23:39-48.

Morahan-Martin J, Schumacher P. Incidence and correlates of pathological Internet use among college students. Comput Hum Behav 2000; 16:13-29.

Ohannessian CM. Does technology use moderate the relationship between parental alcoholism and adolescent alcohol and cigarette use? Addict Behav 2009; 34:606-609.

Orzack MH, Voluse AC, Wolf D, Hennen J. An ongoing study of group treatment for men involved in problematic Internet-enabled sexual behavior. Cyberpsychol Behav 2006; 9:348-360.

Robin-Marie Shepherd RM, Edelmann RJ. Reasons for internet use and social anxiety. Pers Indiv Differ 2005; 39:949-958.

Rollnick S, Mason P, Butler C, Health Behavior Change: A Guide for Practitioners. Elsevier Health Sciences, London: Churchill Livingstone 1999.

Saunders PL, Chester A. Shyness and the internet: Social problem or panacea? Comput Hum Behav 2008; 24:2649-2658.

Shapira NA, Goldsmith TD, Keck PE Jr, Khosla UM, McElroy SL. Psychiatric features of individuals with problematic internet use. J Affect Disord 2000; 57:267-272.

Shapira NA, Lessig MC, Goldsmith TD, Szabo ST, Lazoritz M, Gold MS et al. Problematic internet use: proposed classification and diagnostic criteria. Depress Anxiety 2003; 17:207-216.

Shaw M, Black DW. Internet addiction: definition, assessment, epidemiology and clinical management. CNS Drugs 2008; 22:353-365.

Shek DT, Tang VM, Lo CY. Evaluation of an Internet addiction treatment program for Chinese adolescents in Hong Kong. Adolescence 2009; 44:359-373.

Spada MM, Langston B, Nikcevic AV, Moneta GB. The role of metacognition in problematic internet use. Comput Human Behav 2008; 24:2325-2335.

Petersen KU, Weymann N, Schelb Y, Thiel R, Thomasius R. Pathological Internet use--epidemiology, diagnostics, co-occurring disorders and treatment. Fortschr Neurol Psychiatr 2009; 77:263-271.

Tsai HF, Cheng SH, Yeh TL, Shih CC, Chen KC, Yang YC et al. The risk factors of Internet addiction-a survey of university freshmen. Psychiatr Res 2009; 167:294-299.

Twohig MP, Crosby JM. Acceptance and commitment therapy as a treatment for problematic internet pornography viewing. Behav Ther 2010; 41:285-295. Epub 2010.

Wells A, Cartwright-Hatton S. A short form of the metacognitions questionnaire: Properties of the MCQ-30. Behav Res Ther 2004; 42:385-396.

Whang LS, Lee S, Chang G. Internet over-users' psychological profiles: a behavior sampling analysis on Internet addiction. Cyberpsychol Behav 2003; 6:143-150.

Whitty MT, Carr A. Taking the good with the bad. J Couple Relatsh Ther 2005; 4:103-115.

Widyanto L, Griffiths M. Internet addiction: Does it really exist? (revisited). J Gackenbach (Ed.), Psychology and the Internet: Intrapersonal, Interpersonal, and Transpersonal Implications. Second ed., San Diego, CA, Academic Press, 2007, p.141-163.

Widyanto L, McMurran M. The psychometric properties of the internet addiction test. Cyberpsychol Behav 2004; 7:443-450.

Yen JY, Ko CH, Yen CF, Wu HY, Yang MJ. The comorbid psychiatric symptoms of Internet addiction: attention deficit and hyperactivity disorder (ADHD), depression, social phobia, and hostility. J Adolesc Health 2007; 41:93-98 Epub 2007.

Yoo HJ, Cho SC, Ha J, Yune SK, Kim SJ, Hwang J, Chung A, Sung YH, Lyoo IK. Attention deficit and hyperactivity symptoms and internet addiction. Psychiatry Clin Neurosci 2004; 58:487-494.

Young KS. Caught in the Net: How to Recognize Internet Addiction and A Winning Strategy for Recovery. New York, NY, John Wiley & Sons, Inc., 1998b.

Young KS. Cognitive behavior therapy with internet addicts: treatment outcomes and implications. Cyber-psychol Behav 2007; 10:671-679.

Young KS. Internet addiction: symptoms, evaluations and treatment. In Innovations in Clinical Practice: A Source Book. Edited by VandeCreek L, Jackson TL. Sarasota, FL: Professional Resource Press, 1999, p.19-31. Available at http://www.netaddiction.com/articles/symptoms.pdf (17.06.2009)

Young KS. Internet addiction: the emergence of a new clinical disorder. Cyberpsychol Behav 1998; 1: 237-244.

Young KS, Pistner M, O'Mara J, Buchanan J. Cyber disorders: The mental health concern for the new millennium. Cyberpsychol Behav 1999; 2:475-479.

Young KS. Treating the Internet Addicted Employee. Journal of Employee Assistance 2004; 4:17-18.

Zhou Y, Lin FC, Du YS, Qin LD, Zhao ZM, Xu JR, Lei H. Gray matter abnormalities in Internet addiction: A voxel-based morphometry study. Eur J Radiol Epub 2009.

Permissions

The contributors of this book come from diverse backgrounds, making this book a truly international effort. This book will bring forth new frontiers with its revolutionizing research information and detailed analysis of the nascent developments around the world.

We would like to thank Irismar Reis de Oliveira, for lending his expertise to make the book truly unique. He has played a crucial role in the development of this book. Without his invaluable contribution this book wouldn't have been possible. He has made vital efforts to compile up to date information on the varied aspects of this subject to make this book a valuable addition to the collection of many professionals and students.

This book was conceptualized with the vision of imparting up-to-date information and advanced data in this field. To ensure the same, a matchless editorial board was set up. Every individual on the board went through rigorous rounds of assessment to prove their worth. After which they invested a large part of their time researching and compiling the most relevant data for our readers. Conferences and sessions were held from time to time between the editorial board and the contributing authors to present the data in the most comprehensible form. The editorial team has worked tirelessly to provide valuable and valid information to help people across the globe.

Every chapter published in this book has been scrutinized by our experts. Their significance has been extensively debated. The topics covered herein carry significant findings which will fuel the growth of the discipline. They may even be implemented as practical applications or may be referred to as a beginning point for another development. Chapters in this book were first published by InTech; hereby published with permission under the Creative Commons Attribution License or equivalent.

The editorial board has been involved in producing this book since its inception. They have spent rigorous hours researching and exploring the diverse topics which have resulted in the successful publishing of this book. They have passed on their knowledge of decades through this book. To expedite this challenging task, the publisher supported the team at every step. A small team of assistant editors was also appointed to further simplify the editing procedure and attain best results for the readers.

Our editorial team has been hand-picked from every corner of the world. Their multi-ethnicity adds dynamic inputs to the discussions which result in innovative outcomes. These outcomes are then further discussed with the researchers and contributors who give their valuable feedback and opinion regarding the same. The feedback is then collaborated with the researches and they are edited in a comprehensive manner to aid the understanding of the subject.

Apart from the editorial board, the designing team has also invested a significant amount of their time in understanding the subject and creating the most relevant covers. They scrutinized every image to scout for the most suitable representation of the subject and create an appropriate cover for the book.

The publishing team has been involved in this book since its early stages. They were actively engaged in every process, be it collecting the data, connecting with the contributors or procuring relevant information. The team has been an ardent support to the editorial, designing and production team. Their endless efforts to recruit the best for this project, has resulted in the accomplishment of this book. They are a veteran in the field of academics and their pool of knowledge is as vast as their experience in printing. Their expertise and guidance has proved useful at every step. Their uncompromising quality standards have made this book an exceptional effort. Their encouragement from time to time has been an inspiration for everyone.

The publisher and the editorial board hope that this book will prove to be a valuable piece of knowledge for researchers, students, practitioners and scholars across the globe.

List of Contributors

Irismar Reis de Oliveira
Department of Neurosciences and Mental Health, Federal University of Bahia, Brazil

Amy Wenzel
Wenzel Consulting, LLC, Department of Psychiatry, University of Pennsylvania, USA

Neander Abreu
Institute of Psychology, Federal University of Bahia, Salvador, Brazil

Vania Bitencourt Powell
Post-Graduation Program, Department of Neuroscience and Mental Health, Professor Edgard Santos University Hospital, Federal University of Bahia, Salvador, Brazil

Donna Sudak
Department of Psychiatry, Drexel University, Philadelphia, USA

Robert L. Woolfolk
Rutgers University, USA
Princeton University, USA

Lesley A. Allen
Princeton University, USA
UMDNJ – Robert Wood Johnson Medical School, USA

Mario Francisco P. Juruena
Department of Neurosciences and Behaviour, Faculty of Medicine Ribeirao Preto, University of Sao Paulo, Brazil
Department Psychological Medicine, Institute of Psychiatry, King's College London, U.K.

Aristides V. Cordioli and Analise Vivan
Federal University of Rio Grande do Sul, Porto Alegre, Brazil

Bernard P. Rangé
Graduate Program in Psychology, Psychology Institute, Federal University at Rio de Janeiro, Brazil

Ana Carolina Robbe Mathias
Psychiatric Institute, Federal University at Rio de Janeiro, Brazil

Fugen Neziroglu and Lauren M. Mancusi
Bio-Behavioral Institute, Great Neck, NY, USA

Ömer Şenormancı and Ramazan Konkan
Bakırkoy Research and Training Hospital for Psychiatry, Neurology and Neurosurgery, Turkey

Mehmet Zihni Sungur
Marmara University School of Medicine, Turkey

Printed in the USA
CPSIA information can be obtained
at www.ICGtesting.com
JSHW011400221024
72173JS00003B/363

9 781632 413666